O9-BUC-604

THE

COCONUT
OIL

MIRACLE

THE
COCONUT
OIL
MIRACLE

BRUCE FIFE, C.N., N.D.

Previously published as *The Healing Miracles of Coconut Oil*

AVERY · A MEMBER OF PENGUIN GROUP (USA) INC. · NEW YORK

Every effort has been made to ensure that the information contained in this book is complete and accurate. However, neither the publisher nor the author is engaged in rendering professional advice or services to the individual reader. The ideas, procedures, and suggestions contained in this book are not intended as a substitute for consulting with your physician. All matters regarding your health require medical supervision. Neither the author nor the publisher shall be liable or responsible for any loss or damage allegedly arising from any information or suggestion in this book.

The recipes contained in this book are to be followed exactly as written. The publisher is not responsible for your specific health or allergy needs that may require medical supervision. The publisher is not responsible for any adverse reactions to the recipes contained in this book.

While the author has made every effort to provide accurate telephone numbers and Internet addresses at the time of publication, neither the publisher nor the author assumes any responsibility for errors or for changes that occur after publication.

Most Avery books are available at special quantity discounts for bulk purchase for sales promotions, premiums, fund-raising, and educational needs. Special books or book excerpts also can be created to fit specific needs. For details, write Penguin Group (USA) Inc. Special Markets, 375 Hudson Street, New York, NY 10014.

a member of
Penguin Group (USA) Inc.
375 Hudson Street
New York, NY 10014

Copyright © 1999, 2000, 2002, 2004 by Bruce Fife
Previously published as *The Healing Miracles of Coconut Oil* by Piccadilly Books
All rights reserved. No part of this book may be reproduced, scanned, or distributed in any printed or electronic form without permission. Please do not participate in or encourage piracy of copyrighted materials in violation of the author's rights. Purchase only authorized editions.
Published simultaneously in Canada

Library of Congress Cataloging-in-Publication Data

Fife, Bruce, date.
The coconut oil miracle / Bruce Fife.—[Rev. ed.]
p.   cm.
Rev. ed of: The healing miracles of coconut oil. 2001.
Includes bibliographical references and index.
ISBN 1-58333-204-9
1. Coconut oil—Health aspects.   2. Coconut oil—Therapeutic use.   3. Fatty acids in human nutrition.   I. Fife, Bruce, 1952– Healing miracles of coconut oil.   II. Title.
QP752.F35F545   2004   2004046256
615'.3245—dc22

Printed in the United States of America
20 19 18 17 16 15 14

BOOK DESIGN BY MEIGHAN CAVANAUGH

CONTENTS

• FOREWORD

Up until now only a small group of lipid (fat) researchers were familiar with the incredible health benefits of a unique group of saturated fats found in coconut oil. Most of those in the health care industry have been generally ignorant of these benefits, shunning coconut oil because of common misconceptions regarding dietary fat. But this situation is beginning to change as the amazing nutritional and therapeutic benefits of the tropical oils become better known.

In this book the reader will learn that not all saturated fats are unhealthy. In fact, there is a subgroup of saturated fats that actually have a positive effect on your health. This book provides a brief summary of the remarkable health benefits lipid researchers have slowly been uncovering regarding a unique group of saturated fats found in mother's milk and coconut oil known as "medium-chain fatty acids." The story is fascinating and can have a pronounced effect on your health.

Those who take the time to pick up this book may be surprised to learn that these saturated fats promote good health. Contrary to what is generally believed by both the lay public and medical professionals, the saturated fats found in coconut oil are actually good for you. This should not be surprising, because if coconut oil were unhealthy it would have been evidenced in populations who have used it for generations.

In fact, just the opposite is the case. Those populations who use coconut oil demonstrate a remarkable level of good health.

Historically, coconut oil is one of the earliest oils to be used as a food and as a pharmaceutical. Ayurvedic literature has long promoted the health and cosmetic benefits of coconut oil. Even today the Asian Pacific community, which may represent as much as half the world's population, uses coconut oil in one form or another. Many of these people enjoy remarkably good health and longevity. Studies on people who live in tropical climates and who have a diet high in coconut oil show that they are healthier and have fewer incidences of heart disease, cancer, digestive complaints, and prostate problems. In North America and Europe popular cookbooks from the late nineteenth century often included coconut oil in many recipes, yet heart disease and cancer were almost unheard of at the time. Common sense would suggest that the saturated fats in coconut oil are not the poisons they are often made out to be.

Why, then, all the negative publicity regarding coconut oil? Since it is thought that "saturated fats" are involved in heart disease, coconut oil has been considered a health risk. Much of the information linking coconut oil and increased heart disease is, however, circumstantial at best and flawed at worst. Studies showing that dietary coconut oil raises blood cholesterol and increases the possible risk of heart disease were poorly conceived because the essential fats were not included in the diet. Populations with high levels of coconut oil consumption always include other oils from vegetables and fish for a more balanced diet.

Both "scientific" and political propaganda by the American Soybean Association and the Center for Science in the Public Interest (or is it their own?) have joined forces in a campaign to replace tropical oils with polyunsaturated soybean oil from American farmers. Because of this campaign, food processors and restaurant and theater chains have switched from coconut to polyunsaturated oils. Even dietetic and medical spokespersons, blinded by negative publicity, have supported the switch to polyunsaturated oils as heart healthy. This campaign has condemned all saturated fats as generically "poison." Both the lay and scientific press fail to mention the fact that certain subgroups of saturated fats have positive health benefits.

The abundance of documented scientific facts reviewed for this book will tell, as Paul Harvey would say, "the rest of the story." As the story unfolds, the reader can better appreciate the fact that "saturated fats" are classified into two primary categories: (1) long-chain fats and (2) short- and medium-chain fats. Each subgroup has markedly different biological effects. It will be shown that the overconsumption of polyunsaturated fats in our diet is more detrimental to our health than the saturated fats found in tropical oils.

Not only is coconut oil not a "dietary poison," but it contains a remarkable fat called monolaurin. This medium-chain fat, first discovered in my laboratory, represents one of the most exceptional and inspiring groups of fats found in nature. This unique fat, available naturally from mother's milk and coconut oil, is now commercially available as Lauricidin®. Monolaurin (Lauricidin®) is currently being tested in clinical trials as a treatment for genital herpes, hepatitis C, and HIV. Early clinical results have been very promising and show exciting possibilities for an important new weapon in alternative medicine.

Dr. Bruce Fife should be commended for bringing together in this very readable book the positive health benefits of coconut oil and especially monolaurin. The inquiring reader will have a new and more balanced view of the role of fat, and especially saturated fats, in our diet.

JON J. KABARA, PH.D.
Professor Emeritus, Chemistry and Pharmacology
Michigan State University

THE

COCONUT
OIL

MIRACLE

· INTRODUCTION

Some years ago when I was in a meeting with a group of nutritionists, one of the members of the group made the statement
"Coconut oil is good for you." We all gasped in disbelief. *Coconut oil
healthy? Preposterous,* we thought. Everywhere we go we're told how bad
coconut oil is because it is a source of "artery-clogging" saturated fat.
How could coconut oil be good?

She knew we would doubt her statement and explained, "Coconut
oil has been unjustly criticized and is really one of the good fats." She
cited several studies proving to us that it wasn't the evil villain it was
made out to be and that it actually provided many valuable health benefits. I learned that for several decades it has been used in hospital IV solutions to feed critically ill patients and that it is a major component of
baby formula because it provides many of the same nutrients as human
breast milk. I learned that coconut oil could be used to treat a number
of common illnesses and is considered by the Food and Drug Adminis-
tration (FDA) to be a safe, natural food. (It's on the FDA's exclusive
GRAS list, which means it is "generally regarded as safe.")

After the meeting I was intrigued. I had learned a lot, but it brought
up many questions that troubled me. For instance, if coconut oil was

good, why is it so often portrayed as being unhealthy? If the health benefits are for real, why haven't we heard of them before? Why don't we hear about the use of coconut oil in hospitals, baby formula, and elsewhere? If it's good for the sick and the very young, why wouldn't it be good for us as well? Why would the government include it on its list of safe foods if it were dangerous or unhealthy? Why aren't the studies on coconut oil better publicized? Why have we been misled . . . or have we? Perhaps coconut oil is bad, and hospital patients and parents of formula-fed babies are being deceived. These and many more questions filled my mind. I had to find the answers.

I began a search to find out anything and everything I could about coconut oil. The first thing I discovered was that very little has been written about coconut oil in magazines and books. Even my nutritional textbooks were relatively silent on the subject. No one seemed to know much about it. Almost everything I came across in the "popular" health literature was critical, stating that coconut oil is bad because it is high in saturated fat. Each author seemed to parrot the others, giving no further explanation. It was almost like a royal decree had been sent out to all authors stating that they must say the exact same thing about coconut oil in order to be politically correct (but not necessarily accurate). Saying anything different was against the rules, and that was that. I did find a few—a very few—authors who stood up to this rhetoric and stated bluntly that coconut oil wasn't bad, but they didn't give much detail either. It seemed that nobody really knew anything about it.

The only place I could find cold, hard facts was in often-ignored research journals. Here I found a gold mine of information, and the answers to all my questions. This was the best place for me to search, because these journals report the actual results of studies and are not simply people's opinions, as is most of the material in popular magazines and books. There were literally hundreds of studies published in dozens of the most respected scientific and medical journals. What I learned was absolutely amazing. I found out that coconut oil is one of the most remarkable health foods available. I felt as if I had rediscovered an ancient health food that the world had almost forgotten about. I also learned why coconut oil has been maligned and misunderstood (I will get to that later, and the answer may shock and even anger you).

I started using coconut oil myself and began recommending it to my clients (I am a certified nutritionist and naturopathic physician). I've seen it get rid of chronic psoriasis, eliminate dandruff, remove precancerous skin lesions, speed recovery from the flu, stop bladder infections, overcome chronic fatigue, and relieve hemorrhoids, among other things. In addition to this, the scientific literature reports its possible use in treating dental caries (cavities), peptic ulcers, benign prostatic hyperplasia (enlarged prostate), epilepsy, genital herpes, hepatitis C, and HIV/ AIDS. Yes, as incredible as it sounds, I learned that coconut oil can be used to fight AIDS—a dreadful disease that has been considered incurable! Many AIDS patients have already benefited. Another remarkable benefit of coconut oil is its ability to prevent heart disease. Yes, I said *prevent* heart disease. While for years we've been led to believe that coconut oil promotes this condition, recent research proves otherwise. In fact, in the near future it may gain wide acceptance as a powerful aid in the fight against heart and other cardiovascular diseases.

I've continued to research coconut and other oils. I've been so impressed with the potential health benefits available from coconut oil that I felt an obligation to share what I've learned with the rest of the world. That's why I've written this book. Before I go any further, let me state right here that I do *not* sell coconut oil or have any financial interest in the coconut industry. My purpose in writing this book is to dispel myths and misconceptions and reveal to you some of the many healing miracles of coconut oil. What you will learn in this book may sound incredible, at times maybe even too incredible, but I didn't make this stuff up. Every statement I make in this book is verified by published scientific studies, historical records, and personal experience. If you want to check them out, references and additional resources are listed in the back of this book.

Whenever I talk about coconut oil, the first thing people think is "Isn't that bad for you?" This may have been your reaction when you first saw this book. Stop and think about it for a minute. All you need to do is use a little common sense, and you will see how ridiculous it is to think of coconut oil as being harmful. Coconuts (and coconut oil) have been used as a major source of food for thousands of years by millions of people in Asia, the Pacific Islands, Africa, and Central America. Traditionally these people have had much better health than those in North America and Europe who don't eat coconut. Before the introduction of modern foods, many of these people depended almost entirely on coconut to sustain life. They didn't suffer from heart disease, cancer, arthritis, diabetes, and other modern degenerative diseases, at least not until they abandoned their traditional coconut-based diet and began eating modern foods. It should be, or soon will become, obvious to you that coconut oil isn't the evil villain it has been generally considered to be.

1

THE TRUTH ABOUT
COCONUT OIL

If you were to travel the world looking for a people who enjoy a degree of health far above that found in most nations, a people who are relatively free from the crippling effects of degenerative disease, you couldn't help but be impressed by the natives who inhabit the islands of the South Pacific. These people in their tropical paradise enjoy a remarkable degree of good health, relatively free from the aches and pains of degenerative disease that plague most of the rest of the world. These people are robust and healthy. Heart disease, cancer, diabetes, and arthritis are almost unheard-of—at least among those who continue to live on the traditional native diets.

Researchers have long noted that when these island people start to abandon their traditional diets in favor of Western foods, their health deteriorates. The more westernized the people become, the more their diseases mimic those commonly found in the West. Ian Prior, M.D., a cardiologist and director of the epidemiology unit at the Wellington Hospital in New Zealand, says this pattern has been very clearly demonstrated by Pacific Islanders, and that the further the Pacific natives move away from the diet of their ancestors, the more frequently they experience degenerative disease such as gout, diabetes, atherosclerosis, obesity, and hypertension.

What is the miracle food these people eat that protects them from degenerative disease? What is this mysterious food that has been used throughout the tropical island cultures in the Pacific yet is relatively uncommon in Western diets? A survey of the types of foods common among these people would include bananas, mangoes, papayas, kiwi, taro, sego palm root, and coconut. While all of these are common in the tropics, only a few are widely dispersed and used as staple food sources by millions of island inhabitants. Mangoes, for example, are found only in limited locations and are not an important food source in most island populations. Bananas, likewise, are abundant in some areas but relatively rare in others and do not contribute much, if at all, to the diets of the people in other localities.

The most universally eaten foods among the Polynesian and Asian communities around the Pacific are the roots of the taro and sego palm and the fruit of the coconut tree. Taro and sego palm roots are rich sources of fiber and carbohydrate and form the staple diet of many island populations, much as rice or wheat do in other parts of the world. Nutritionally, however, these foods are inferior to rice and wheat, containing fewer vitamins and minerals per volume. Such foods could hardly be the secret of the islanders' good health.

The only other food eaten universally throughout the area is the coconut. Coconuts have been used as a staple part of the diets of almost all Polynesian and Melanesian and many Asian peoples in this area for centuries. They are used as food and as flavoring and are made into beverages. They are highly prized for their rich oil content, which is used for all cooking purposes.

Coconut oil has a long and highly respected reputation in many cultures throughout the world, not only as a valuable food but also as an effective medicine. It is used throughout the tropics in many of the traditional systems of medicine. For example, in India it is an important ingredient in some of the ayurvedic medical formulations. Ayurvedic medicine has been practiced in India for thousands of years and is still used as the primary form of medical treatment by millions of people. In the Central American country of Panama, people are known to drink coconut oil by the glass to help themselves overcome sickness. They have learned over the generations that consuming coconut oil speeds recovery from illness. In Jamaica, coconut is considered a health tonic good for the heart. In Nigeria and other parts of tropical Africa, palm kernel oil (which is very similar to coconut oil) is a trusted remedy for all types of illnesses. It has been used there with success for so long that it is the most commonly administered traditional remedy. Among the Polynesian people the coconut palm is valued above all other plants for its nutritional and health-giving properties. The healing miracles of the coconut have long been recognized in those cultures where it is grown. Only recently have these benefits started to become known to the rest of the world.

While still widely unknown to Western society, the therapeutic benefits of the unique oil found in coconuts are well known among lipid (oil) researchers. This oil is used in hospitals to feed patients who have digestive or malabsorption problems. It is commonly given to infants and small children who cannot digest other fats. It has been a primary ingredient in most commercial infant formulas. Unlike other fats, coconut oil protects against heart disease, cancer, diabetes, and a host of other degenerative illnesses. It supports and strengthens the immune system, thus helping the body ward off attack from infection and disease. It is unique among oils in that it promotes weight loss, which has earned it the reputation of being the world's only low-calorie fat.

In our modern society, where we are constantly being advised to reduce fat intake, it sounds strange to learn that eating any one particular type of oil can be healthy and actually prevent disease. But eating more oil may be one of the healthiest dietary changes you can make—if it's coconut oil. We are told that in order to reduce the risk of heart disease we should limit fat consumption to no more than 30 percent of our total calorie intake per day. However, Polynesian peoples consume large quantities of fat, primarily from coconut. For some, fat makes up as much as 60 percent of their total calorie intake—twice the limit recommended as prudent. The 30 percent limit is probably a good standard with oils typically eaten in Western countries, but coconut oil is different. It is one of the "good" oils that promotes better health. As researchers have studied coconut oil, it has emerged as the premiere dietary oil of all time, providing health benefits that surpass even those of other highly regarded oils.

Whenever coconut oil is mentioned, most people immediately think of saturated fat and therefore assume it must be bad. It's true that coconut oil is primarily a saturated fat. What people don't realize, however, is that there are many different types of saturated fat and all of them affect the body differently. The type of saturated fat found in coconut oil, a plant source, is different from the type found in animal products. The difference is dramatic and is fully documented by years of scientific research.

If you've been avoiding coconut oil because of its saturated fat content, you are among hundreds of thousands of others who have been purposely misled by self-serving commercial enterprises. At this point, you may be skeptical and perhaps even resistant to the idea that coconut oil can be healthy. At one time I felt the same way. But several years of intensive research into the scientific literature as well as firsthand clinical use have revealed a new image of this marvelous dietary oil. Much of the information presented in this book is so new that even most health care professionals aren't aware of it yet.

Using coconut oil for all your cooking needs may be one of the healthiest decisions you could ever make. In this book you will discover many of the health-promoting benefits coconuts and coconut oil can bring to you. You will also learn why many researchers now consider coconut oil to be the healthiest oil on earth. You will discover why many Asian and Polynesian people call the coconut palm the "Tree of Life."

THE TROPICAL OILS WAR

At this point you may be asking: "If coconut oil is as good as you say it is, why has it had such a bad reputation?" The simple reason is money, politics, and misunderstanding. Everybody knows coconut oil is a saturated fat, and we're constantly told to reduce our saturated fat intake. The words "saturated fat" have become almost synonymous with "heart disease." Very few people know the difference between the medium-chain saturated fatty acids in coconut oil and the long-chain saturated fatty acids in meat and other foods. To most people, saturated fat is saturated fat—an evil substance lurking in foods waiting for the opportunity to attack and strike you down with a heart attack. Even medical professionals don't know there is a difference. Most don't even know there is more than one type of saturated fat (the different types are discussed in the next chapter). Unfortunately, many health care workers and health and fitness writers only repeat what they hear and have no understanding of fats and how they affect the body. Only recently has the truth about coconut oil been reemerging.

As far back as the 1950s, research began to show the health benefits of coconut oil. For many years it was considered a good oil with many nutritional uses. So how did coconut oil become a despised, artery-clogging villain? Much of the credit goes to the American Soybean Association (ASA). It began in the mid-1980s. At the time, the media were stirred into a frenzy, warning the public about a newly discovered health threat—tropical oils. Coconut oil, they proclaimed, was a saturated fat and would cause heart attacks. Everywhere you turned, any product that contained coconut or palm oil was criticized as being "unhealthful." In response to the seemingly overwhelming public response, movie theaters began cooking their popcorn in soybean oil; food makers began switching from the tropical oils they had used for years to soybean oil; restaurants stopped using tropical oils in favor of soybean and other vegetable oils. By the early 1990s, the tropical oils market had dwindled to a fraction of what it once was. The promoters of this media blitz declared a victory in their fight against tropical oils.

This war of oils, unfortunately, made every man, woman, and child in America (and elsewhere) its victim. Tragically, the oil that replaced coconut and palm oils was hydrogenated vegetable oil (principally from soybeans)—one of the most health-damaging dietary oils in existence—

and the only people who actually benefited from this new health craze were those in the soybean industry. These hydrogenated replacements contain as much saturated fat as the tropical oils, but they are not made from easily digested medium-chain fatty acids like those found in coconut oil—they are composed of toxic trans fatty acids. The result has been to replace healthy tropical oils with some very nasty, chemically altered vegetable oils. We are all victims, because when we eat foods containing these oils our health suffers.

The entire campaign was a carefully orchestrated plan by the ASA to eliminate competition from imported tropical oils. During the 1960s and 1970s, research indicated that some forms of saturated fat increase blood cholesterol. Since elevated cholesterol is recognized as a risk factor in the development of heart disease, saturated fat was, consequently, regarded as an undesirable food component, and we were advised to reduce our intake of it. The prevailing opinion was that the less saturated fat you ate, the better.

Capitalizing on the public's fear of saturated fat and its perceived association with heart disease, the ASA set out to create a health crisis. The crisis they planned would be so terrifying it would literally scare people away from using tropical oils. In 1986 the ASA sent a "Fat Fighter Kit" to soybean farmers encouraging them to write government officials, food companies, and so on, protesting the encroachment of "highly saturated tropical fats like palm and coconut oils." The wives and families of some 400,000 soybean growers were encouraged to fan out across the country in a lobbying effort touting the health benefits of soybean oil. Well-meaning but misguided health groups such as the Center for Science in the Public Interest (CSPI) joined in the battle, issuing news releases referring to palm, coconut, and palm kernel oils as "artery-clogging fats."

The CSPI, a nonprofit consumer activist group, had been criticizing saturated fats since its founding in the 1970s. Like most nutrition advocates at the time, they mistakenly believed that all saturated fats were the same and attacked them with a vengeance. Encouraged by the publicity generated by the ASA, they began to intensify their attack. The tropical oils, being highly saturated, were severely criticized in their promotional literature, news releases, and lobbying efforts. It seemed the CSPI considered saturated fat to be the worst evil ever to beset humankind. The ASA had found a powerful, vocal ally in its campaign to take over the tropical oils market.

For a group that claimed to be an advocate for responsible nutritional education, the CSPI was surprisingly ignorant regarding saturated fats, especially concerning coconut oil. Instead of informing the public about the truth regarding saturated fats, they only succeeded in strengthening misconceptions and falsehoods. The CSPI's lack of knowledge concerning lipid biochemistry is revealed in a booklet they published called *Saturated Fat Attack*. While laypeople and many health care professionals may have been fooled by the information in this booklet, nutritional biochemist Mary G. Enig, Ph.D., says, "There were lots of substantive mistakes in the booklet, including errors in the description of the biochemistry of fats and oils and completely erroneous statements about the fat and oil composition of many of the products." Most people, however, would not have known this, and the booklet and other inaccurate information distributed by the group succeeded in convincing many to completely shun tropical oils. The CSPI's lack of accurate scientific knowledge made them an unsuspecting puppet for the ASA.

In October 1988, the Nebraska millionaire Phil Sokolof, a recovered heart attack patient and founder of the National Heart Savers Association, jumped on the media bandwagon. He began running full-page newspaper advertisements accusing food companies of "poisoning America" by using tropical oils with high levels of saturated fat. Radically anti–saturated fat, he staged a blistering national ad campaign attacking tropical oils as a health danger. One ad showed a coconut "bomb" with a lighted wick and cautioned consumers that their health was threatened by coconut and palm oils. Before long, everybody believed that coconut oil caused heart disease.

Food manufacturers joined in too. Hoping to profit from the anti–tropical oils sentiment, they tried to add labels to their products that read "contains no tropical oil." The Federal Trade Commission (FTC) ruled such labels illegal because the statement implied a health claim, which portrayed the product as being better for not having tropical oil, and there was no evidence to back it up.

FICTION TRIUMPHS OVER FACT

Meanwhile, tropical oil exporters from Malaysia prepared a public relations campaign against what it called "vicious scare tactics" being used against its product. The tropical oil war was in full swing. At stake was the $3-billion-a-year vegetable oil market in the United States, where the dominant domestic soy oil producers had launched a vicious propaganda war against foreign competitors. The tropical oil industry, having few allies and comparatively little financial muscle to retaliate, couldn't match the combined efforts of the ASA, the CSPI, and others. Few would listen to the lone voices protesting the dissemination of the false information attacking tropical oils.

When the attack on coconut oil began, those medical and research professionals who were familiar with it wondered why. They knew coconut oil did not contribute to heart disease and that it provided many health advantages. Some even stepped forward to set the record straight. But by this time public sentiment had firmly sided with the ASA, and people refused to listen.

Researchers familiar with tropical oils were called on to testify at Senate hearings on the health implications of these products. "Coconut oil has a neutral effect on blood cholesterol, even in situations where coconut oil is the sole source of fat," reported Dr. George Blackburn, a Harvard Medical School researcher who testified at a congressional hearing about tropical oils held on June 21, 1988. "These (tropical) oils have been consumed as a substantial part of the diet of many groups for thousands of years with absolutely no evidence of any harmful effects to the populations consuming them," said Mary G. Enig, Ph.D., an expert on fats and oils and a former research associate at the University of Maryland.

Dr. C. Everett Koop, former surgeon general of the United States, called the tropical oil scare "foolishness." Commercial interests either trying to divert blame to others or ignorantly following the saturated-fat hysteria were "terrorizing the public about nothing." Dr. David Klurfeld, chairman of the Department of Nutrition and Food Science at Wayne State University, called the anti–tropical oils campaign "public relations mumbo jumbo." He pointed out that tropical oils amounted to only about 2 percent of the American diet and that even if they were as bad as the ASA claimed, they wouldn't have much of an effect on health: "The amount of tropical oils in the U.S. diet is so low that there is no reason to worry about it. The countries with the highest palm oil intakes in the world are Costa Rica and Malaysia. Their heart disease rates and serum cholesterol levels are much lower than in western nations. This [tropical oils scare] never was a real health issue."

Despite testimonials of respected medical professionals and lipid researchers, the media paid little attention. The saturated-fat crisis was news, and that got headlines. Major newspapers and television and radio networks picked up the anti–saturated-fat ads and developed alarming news stories. One such story was titled "The Oil from Hell." Those who knew the truth about coconut oil were ignored and even criticized by those brainwashed by the media blitz. Because of the frenzy stirred up by the ASA and their friends, the fictional message they trumpeted won out over scientific fact.

CURSE OF THE TRANS FATTY ACIDS

Catering to public sentiment, McDonald's, Burger King, and Wendy's restaurants announced they would replace the saturated fat they had been using with more "healthful" vegetable oils. The switch to the new vegetable oils actually increased the fat content of the fried foods—hardly a healthful move. Tests by the FDA and others found that french fries cooked in beef tallow absorb less fat than those cooked in vegetable oil, which led to estimates that the switch to vegetable oil would more than double the fat content of fries and increase fat consumption. In addition, the fat was hydrogenated. This kind of fat is worse than beef tallow because it contains toxic trans fatty acids. Trans fatty acids have a greater negative effect on blood cholesterol than beef tallow and therefore are considered to carry a greater risk for heart disease.

The ASA succeeded in producing a health crisis where none had existed. The general ignorance about nutrition by most people swayed them into siding with the soybean industry, which proves that money and politics can override truth. In reality, there was no public outcry; the change was mainly brought about by an aggressive negative campaign. As a result, most major food companies, sensitive to consumer fear, reformulated hundreds of products, replacing tropical oils with hydrogenated oils. Since 1990, the fast food industry has been cooking french fries in hydrogenated vegetable oil instead of beef tallow and tropical oils. They made the change because of the prevailing opinion that vegetable oils were healthier than other oils.

Breads, cookies, crackers, soups, stews, sauces, candy, and frozen and prepared foods of all sorts typically had been made using tropical oils. Up until the late 1980s, tropical oils were common ingredients in many of our foods. They were used extensively by the food industry because they gave foods many desirable properties. These plant-derived saturated fats, being highly stable, do not go rancid, as polyunsaturated oils do. When tropical oils were used, foods remained fresh longer and were better for you. That's not the case any more. It's hard to find foods made with tropical oils nowadays.

As a result of the tropical oils war, coconut and palm oils have nearly disappeared from our food supply. The consequence is that we now consume far less of the health-promoting fatty acids found in coconut oil and much more of the health-destroying trans fatty acids found in hydrogenated soybean oil. Nearly 80 percent of all the vegetable oil used in the United States today comes from soybeans. Three-fourths of that oil is hydrogenated (containing up to 50 percent trans fatty acids). This amounts to an awful lot of nasty trans fatty acids that are in our foods now that weren't there before. For example, a single restaurant meal that in 1982 contained only 2.4 grams of trans fatty acids contains a whopping 19.2 grams of them today. The food is the same; only the oil is different. Because hydrogenated oils are used everywhere, we are cursed with trans fatty acids just about anytime we eat (unless we prepare our food from scratch).

Yes, we lost the war. We lost the many health benefits that can result from regular consumption of coconut products. And we gained too. We gained an increased chance of suffering from heart disease, cancer, diabetes, infectious disease, obesity, and immune dysfunction. These are conditions that have all been tied to the consumption of hydrogenated and partially hydrogenated vegetable oils. Through the cunning marketing strategies of the ASA and the misguided efforts of public interest groups, we have replaced a good health-promoting fat with a very destructive and harmful one.

Even now the cinders of this war still burn. Many ill-informed writers and speakers continue to condemn coconut oil as containing "artery-clogging" saturated fat. But who are you going to believe? Are you going to believe the soybean industry, which has a huge financial interest at stake, or are you going to believe the research based on Pacific Islanders, who eat a great deal of coconut oil and have far better health than the rest of us, and residents of Sri Lanka, who eat lots of coconut oil but have one of the lowest rates of heart disease in the world? Personally, I believe those people who eat coconut oil and don't have heart disease. In Western countries we eat very little coconut oil but consume a significant amount of hydrogenated vegetable oils. The result? Heart disease is on a rampage. It is our number one killer.

Studies have clearly shown that natural coconut oil as a part of a normal diet has a neutral effect on blood cholesterol. Nonhydrogenated, nonadulterated coconut oil has absolutely no adverse health effects. Epidemiological studies show conclusively that populations that consume large amounts of coconut oil experience almost no heart disease, as compared to other populations whose diets contain only a small amount of coconut oil. If coconut oil did have any adverse health effects associated with it, we would see it reflected in the morbidity and mortality in populations that are high consumers of coconut oil. Yet they are among the healthiest people in the world. Simple logic clearly refutes the ASA smear campaign. As you will discover in the following chapters, coconut oil offers so many health benefits it is correctly labeled "the healthiest oil on earth."

2

UNDERSTANDING FATS

In this chapter I describe the differences between saturated and unsaturated fats and explain the reason why coconut oil is different from all the rest. Since the uniqueness of each oil depends on its chemical makeup, I am forced to describe the differences in chemical terms. Unfortunately, when chemistry is discussed it is easy for those people who lack a scientific background to become confused. Please bear with me; I will make my explanation simple enough for the layperson to understand. If you get confused, that's okay, skim through the material and go on to the end chapter. The purpose of this chapter is to provide you with a scientific foundation. You don't need to know chemistry in order to benefit from using coconut oil.

TRIGLYCERIDES AND FATTY ACIDS

Doctors often use the term *lipid* in referring to fat. Lipid is a general term that includes several fatlike compounds in the body. By far the most abundant and the most important of the lipids are the triglycerides. When we speak of fats and oils we are usually referring to triglycerides. Two other lipids—phospholipids and sterols (which include cholesterol)—technically are not fats because they are not triglycerides. But they have similar characteristics and are often referred to as fats.

What is the difference between a fat and an oil? The terms *fat* and *oil* are often used interchangeably. Generally speaking, the only real difference is that fats are considered solid at room temperature while oils remain liquid. Lard, for example, would be referred to as a fat, while corn oil is called an oil. Both, however, are fats.

When you cut into a steak, the white fatty tissue you see is composed of triglycerides (cholesterol is also present, but it is intermingled within the meat fibers and undetectable with the naked eye). The fat that is a nuisance to us, the type that hangs on our arms, looks like jelly on our thighs, and can make your stomach look like a spare tire, is composed of triglycerides. It is the triglycerides that make up our body fat and the fat we see and eat in our foods. About 95 percent of the lipids in our diet, from both plant and animal sources, are triglycerides.

Triglycerides are composed of individual fat molecules known as *fatty acids*. It takes three fatty acid molecules to make a single triglyceride molecule. Fatty acids are linked together by a single glycerol molecule. The glycerol molecule acts as a backbone, so to speak, for the triglyceride.

There are dozens of different types of fatty acids. Scientists have grouped these into three general categories: saturated, monounsaturated, and polyunsaturated. Each category contains several members. So there are many different types of saturated fat, just as there are many types of monounsaturated and polyunsaturated fats.

Each of the fatty acids, regardless of whether it is saturated or not, affects the body differently and exerts different influences on health. Therefore, one saturated fat may have adverse health effects, while another may promote better health. The same is true of monounsaturated and polyunsaturated fats. For example, olive oil has been hailed as one of the "good" fats because those people who eat it in place of other oils have less heart disease. Olive oil is composed primarily of a monounsaturated fatty acid called oleic acid. However, not all monounsaturated fats are healthy. Another monounsaturated fatty acid, known as erucic acid, is extremely toxic to the heart, more so than perhaps any other fatty acid known (Belitz and Grosch). The difference between the two, chemically, is very slight. Likewise, some polyunsaturated fatty acids can also cause problems. On the other hand, the saturated fatty acids that are found in coconut oil have no harmful effects and actually promote better health. So we cannot say one oil is "bad" because it is saturated while another is "good" because it is monounsaturated or polyunsaturated. It all depends on the type of fatty acid and not simply on its degree of saturation.

No dietary oil is purely saturated or unsaturated. All natural fats and oils consist of a mixture of the three classes of fatty acids. To say an oil is saturated or monounsaturated is a gross oversimplification. Olive oil is often called "monounsaturated" because it is *predominantly* monounsaturated, but, like all vegetable oils, it also contains some polyunsaturated and saturated fat as well (see table 2.1 for the amounts of each kind of fatty acid found in different fats and oils).

Table 2.1. Composition of Dietary Fats

FAT	PERCENT OF SATURATED FATS	PERCENT OF MONOUNSATURATED FATS	PERCENT OF POLYUNSATURATED FATS
Canola oil	6	62	32
Safflower oil	10	13	77
Sunflower oil	11	20	69
Corn oil	13	25	62
Soybean oil	15	24	61
Olive oil	14	77	9
Chicken fat	31	47	22
Lard	41	47	12
Beef fat	52	44	4
Palm oil	51	39	10
Butter	66	30	4
Coconut oil	92	6	2

Animal fats are generally the highest in saturated fat. Vegetable oils contain saturated fat as well as monounsaturated and polyunsaturated fat. Most vegetable oils are high in polyunsaturated fats, the exception being palm and coconut oils, which are very high in saturated fat. Coconut oil contains as much as 92 percent saturated fat—more than any other oil, including beef fat and lard.

There are many factors that contribute to the healthfulness of each type of fat—its saturation, the size of the carbon chain, and its susceptibility to peroxidation and free-radical generation.

SATURATION AND SIZE

We hear the terms *saturated, monounsaturated,* and *polyunsaturated* all the time, but what do they mean? What is saturated fat saturated with? How does the degree of saturation affect health? Let me answer those questions. All fatty acids consist primarily of a chain of carbon atoms with varying numbers of hydrogen atoms attached to them. Each carbon atom can hold a maximum of two hydrogen atoms. A fatty acid molecule that has two hydrogen atoms attached to each carbon is said to be "saturated" with hydrogen because it is holding all the hydrogen atoms it possibly can. This type of fatty acid is called a saturated fat. A fatty acid that is missing a pair of hydrogen atoms is called a monounsaturated fat. If more than two hydrogen atoms are missing, it's called a polyunsaturated fat. The more hydrogen atoms are missing, the more polyunsaturated the fat is considered to be.

Wherever a pair of hydrogen atoms is missing, the adjoining carbon atoms must form a double bond (see the illustrations opposite), which produces a weak link in the carbon chain that can have a dramatic influence on health.

The concept of saturation can be described using the analogy of a school bus full of kids. The bus could represent the carbon chain and the students the hydrogen atoms. Each seat on the bus can hold two stu-

```
     H H H H H H H H H H H H H H H H H O
     | | | | | | | | | | | | | | | | | ||
H-C-C-C-C-C-C-C-C-C-C-C-C-C-C-C-C-C-C-O-H
     | | | | | | | | | | | | | | | | |
     H H H H H H H H H H H H H H H H H H
```

Figure 1: Saturated fats are loaded, or saturated, with all the hydrogen (H) atoms they can carry. The example shown above is stearic acid, an 18-carbon saturated fat commonly found in beef fat.

```
     H H H H H H H H         H H H H H H H O
     | | | | | | | |         | | | | | | | ||
H-C-C-C-C-C-C-C-C-C=C-C-C-C-C-C-C-C-C-O-H
     | | | | | | | | | | | | | | | | |
     H H H H H H H H H H H H H H H H H H
```

Figure 2: If one pair of hydrogen atoms were to be removed from the saturated fat, the carbon atoms would form double bonds wtih one another in order to satisfy their bonding requirements. The result would be an unsaturated fat. In this case it would form a monounsaturated fatty acid. The example shown is oleic acid, an 18-chain monounsaturated fatty acid that is found predominantly in olive oil.

```
     H H H H H         H       H H H H H H H O
     | | | | |         |       | | | | | | | ||
H-C-C-C-C-C-C=C-C-C=C-C-C-C-C-C-C-C-C-O-H
     | | | | | | | | | | | | | | | | |
     H H H H H H H H H H H H H H H H H H
```

Figure 3: If two or more pairs of hydrogen atoms are missing and more than one double carbon bond are present, it is referred to as a polyunsaturated oil. The example illustrated is linoleic acid, an 18-chain polyunsaturated acid. This is the most common fat in vegetable oils.

dents, just as each carbon can hold two hydrogen atoms. A bus filled to capacity so there are no empty seats would be analogous to a saturated fat. No more students can fit on the bus. If two students get off the bus and leave one seat vacant, that would be analogous to a monounsaturated fat. If four or more students get off the bus, leaving two or more empty seats, that would be like a polyunsaturated fat. A school bus that is only half filled would be like a fatty acid that is very polyunsaturated.

The length of the fatty acid chain, or size of the school bus, is also important. Some fatty acids contain only two carbon atoms, while others have as many as 24 or more. The two-carbon fatty acid would be like a bus that has only two seats, so that it can carry a maximum of four students—two in each seat. A fatty acid with 24 carbon atoms would be like a long bus with 24 seats, accommodating 48 students.

Acetic acid, found in vinegar, has a chain only two carbon atoms long. A longer acid chain may have four, six, eight, or more carbon atoms. Naturally occurring fatty acids usually occur in even numbers. Butyric acid, one type of fatty acid commonly found in butter, consists of a four-carbon chain. The predominant fatty acids found in meats and fish are 14 or more carbon atoms long. Stearic acid, common in beef fat, has an 18-carbon chain. The 14- to 24-carbon fatty acids are known as long-chain fatty acids (LCFAs). Medium-chain fatty acids (MCFAs) range from 8 to 12 carbons, and short-chain (SCFAs) range from two to six carbons. The length of the carbon chain is a key factor in the way dietary fat is digested and metabolized and how it affects the body.

When three fatty acids of similar length are joined together by a glycerol molecule, the resulting molecule is referred to as a long-chain triglyceride (LCT), medium-chain triglyceride (MCT), or short-chain triglyceride (SCT). You will often see *medium-chain triglyceride* or *MCT* listed as an ingredient on food and supplement labels.

Both the degree of saturation and length of the carbon chain of the fatty acids determine their chemical properties and their effects on our health. The more saturated the fat and the longer the chain, the harder the fat and the higher the melting point. Saturated fat, like that found in lard, is solid at room temperature. Polyunsaturated fat, like corn oil, is liquid at room temperature. Monounsaturated fat is liquid at room temperature, but in the refrigerator it begins to solidify slightly and becomes cloudy or semisolid.

Table 2.2 lists the most common fats found in foods. The fats found in animal tissue, as well as our own bodies, are mainly the triglycerides consisting of stearic, palmitic, and oleic acids. Oleic acid is a monounsaturated fat. Stearic and palmitic acids are saturated fats. The saturated

Table 2.2. Carbons and Double Bonds in Fatty Acids

FATTY ACID	NUMBER OF CARBONS	NUMBER OF DOUBLE BONDS	COMMON SOURCE
SATURATED FATTY ACIDS			
Acetic	2	0	Vinegar
Butyric	4	0	Butterfat
Caproic	6	0	Butterfat
Caprylic	8	0	Coconut oil
Capric	10	0	Palm oil
Lauric	12	0	Coconut oil
Myristic	14	0	Nutmeg oil
Palmitic	16	0	Animal and vegetable oil
Stearic	18	0	Animal and vegetable oil
Arachidic	20	0	Peanut oil
MONOSATURATED FATTY ACIDS			
Palmitoleic	16	1	Butterfat
Oleic	18	1	Olive oil
Erucic	22	1	Rapeseed oil (canola)★
POLYUNSATURATED FATTY ACIDS			
Linoleic	18	2	Vegetable oil
Alpha-lineolenic	18	3	Linseed oil
Arachidonic	20	4	Lecithin
Eicosapentaenoic	20	5	Fish oils
Docosahexaenoic	22	6	Fish oils

★ Rapeseed oil contains as much as 55 percent erucic acid—a very toxic fatty acid. Canola oil in our foods has been genetically altered to include only 1 percent or less erucic acid.

fats found in food consists of a mixture of the different types. Milk, for example contains palmitic, myristic, stearic, lauric, butyric, caproic, caprylic, and capric acids. Each of the fatty acids exerts different effects on the body that are governed by the length of the carbon chain and the degree of unsaturation (number of double bonds).

Saturated fatty acids with up to 26 carbon atoms (C:26) and as few as 2 carbons (C:2) in the chain have been identified as constituents of fats. Of these, palmitic acid (C:16) is the most common, occurring in almost all fats. Myristic (C:14) and stearic (C:18) acids are other common saturated fatty acids.

Short-chain fatty acids (SCFAs) are relatively rare. The most common sources are vinegar and butter. Milk contains tiny amounts of the shorter-chain fatty acids. These fats are concentrated in the making of butter and comprise about 12 percent of its total fat content. Medium-chain fatty acids are also relatively rare but found in moderate concentrations in some tropical nuts and oils.

Long-chain fatty acids are by far the most common fatty acids found in nature. They provide the most efficient or compact energy package and thus make the best storage fats in both plants and animals. Fat cells in our bodies and those of animals are almost entirely long-chained, as are the fats in plants. The vast majority of the fats in our diet are composed of long-chain fatty acids. There are only a few good natural sources of the shorter chain fatty acids. The best source by far is coconut oil.

TROPICAL OILS ARE UNIQUE

Coconut oil and its relatives, the palm and palm kernel oils, are unique in that they are the best natural source of medium- and short-chain fatty acids, giving them their incredible health-promoting properties.

Palm oil contains only a small amount of medium-chain fatty acids. Coconut and palm kernel oils are by far our richest dietary sources of MCFAs: palm kernel oil contains 58 percent MCFAs and coconut oil

64 percent. Because they are both composed predominantly of MCFAs, their effects on health are characterized by the chemical and biological properties associated with these fatty acids.

Most fats in our foods, if not used immediately as an energy source, are stored as fat tissue on our bodies. Coconut oil, being composed primarily of medium- and short-chain fatty acids, has a totally different effect on the body from that of the typical long-chain fatty acids (both saturated and unsaturated) found abundantly in meat and vegetable oils. Medium-chain fatty acids in coconut oil are broken down and used predominately for energy production and thus seldom end up as body fat or as deposits in arteries or anywhere else. They produce energy, not fat. Medium-chain fatty acids do not have a negative effect on blood cholesterol and help protect against heart disease.

FREE RADICALS

Research over the past three decades has identified free radicals as a key player in the cause and development of degenerative disease and aging. Simply put, a free radical is a renegade molecule that has lost an electron in its outer shell, leaving an unpaired electron. This creates a highly unstable and powerful molecular entity. Free radicals will quickly attack and steal an electron from a neighboring molecule. The second molecule, now with one less electron, becomes a highly reactive free radical itself and pulls an electron off yet another nearby molecule. This process continues in a destructive chain reaction that may affect hundreds and even thousands of molecules.

Once a molecule becomes a radical, its physical and chemical properties are permanently changed. When this molecule is part of a living cell, it affects the function of the entire cell. Free radicals can attack our cells, literally ripping their protective membranes apart. Sensitive cellular components like the nucleus and DNA, which carry the genetic blueprint of the cell, can be damaged, leading to cellular mutations and death.

The more free radicals attack our cells, the greater the damage and the greater the potential for serious destruction to vital organs, joints, and bodily systems. Free-radical damage has been linked to the loss of tissue integrity and to physical degeneration. As cells are bombarded by free radicals, the tissues become progressively impaired. Some researchers believe that free-radical destruction is the primary cause of aging. The older the body gets, the more damage it sustains from a lifetime accumulation of attack from free radicals.

Today some 60 or so degenerative diseases are recognized as having free-radical involvement in their cause or manifestation. Additional diseases are regularly being added to this list. Research that linked the major killer diseases such as heart disease and cancer to free radicals has expanded to include atherosclerosis, stroke, varicose veins, hemorrhoids, hypertension, wrinkled skin, dermatitis, arthritis, digestive problems, reproductive problems, cataracts, loss of energy, diabetes, allergies, and failing memory.

We are exposed to free radicals from the pollutants in the air we breathe and from the chemical additives and toxins in the foods we eat and drink. Some free-radical reactions occur as part of the natural process of cellular metabolism. We can't avoid all the free radicals in our environment, but we can limit them. Cigarette smoke, for example, causes free-radical reactions in the lungs. Certain foods and food additives also promote destructive free-radical reactions that affect the entire body. Limiting your exposure to these free-radical–causing substances will reduce your risk of developing a number of degenerative conditions. In this regard, the types of oil you use have a very pronounced effect on your health, because many oils promote the formation of free radicals.

POLYUNSATURATED OILS

When nutritionists tell us to reduce fat intake, we automatically think only of saturated fat. But the recommendation is to reduce all fats, including polyunsaturated fats. In an attempt to reduce saturated fat, people often substitute vegetable oils for those of animal origin. Many vegetable fats, however, are no better than the animal fats we try so hard to avoid. In some cases they can be even worse! The thing that makes vegetable oils potentially harmful is the unsaturation. The double-carbon bonds in the molecule of the polyunsaturated oil are highly vulnerable to oxidation and free-radical formation.

Polyunsaturated oils become toxic when they are oxidized as the result of exposure to oxygen, heat, or light (sunlight or artificial), causing rancidity and the formation of free radicals. Free radicals deplete our antioxidant reserves and cause chemical reactions that damage tissues and cells. When oils are extracted from seeds, they are immediately exposed to oxygen, heat, and light, so the oxidation process starts before the oil even leaves the factory. By the time we buy the oil in the store it has already become rancid to some degree. The more processing an oil undergoes, the more chance it has of oxidizing. The safest vegetable oils to use are those processed at low temperatures and packaged in dark containers. Cold-pressed oils are minimally processed, so they retain most of their natural antioxidants. These antioxidants are important because they retard spoilage by slowing down oxidation and free-radical formation.

Oils are masters of deception. You can't tell a rogue from a saint. They all pretty much look alike. The most toxic vegetable oil can appear as sweet and pure as those that are freshly extracted under ideal conditions. Jurg Loliger, Ph.D., of the Nestle Research Center in Switzerland, says in the authoritative book *Free Radicals and Food Additives* that primary oxidation products of vegetable oils have no objectionable flavor or taste, but the secondary degradation products are generally very potent flavor modifiers and can modify the structure of the product. So pure vegetable oil may be very rancid but give no indication of this because it may not affect its taste or smell. You can eat rancid vegetable oil and not realize it; if mixed with other substances, the free-radical reactions may cause these other substances to produce an unpleasant smell and taste.

While vegetable oils are stored in warehouses, transported in hot trucks, and sit on the store shelves, they are going rancid. They are not refrigerated. They are usually bottled in clear containers where light can penetrate and create more free radicals. These oils may sit around exposed to warm temperatures and light for months before they are sold. But because pure vegetable oil does not produce any noticeable signs of rancidity, we assume them to be safe. All conventionally processed and refined vegetable oils are rancid to some extent by the time they reach the store.

To make matters worse, the vegetable oils we buy sit in our kitchen cupboards for months. And when we use them they are almost always cooked with our food. The cooking accelerates the oxidizing process, making the oil even more rancid and unhealthy. It's ironic that people will buy cold-pressed oil at the health food store and then turn it into a health hazard by cooking with it. Studies show that diets containing heat-treated liquid corn oil were found to produce more atherosclerosis than those containing unheated corn oil. Even a small amount of heated polyunsaturated vegetable oil, especially if eaten frequently over time, will affect your health.

All vegetable oils should be sealed in airtight, opaque containers and stored in the refrigerator. While this won't completely stop free-radical generation, it will slow it down. If you have oils that have not been stored this way, throw them out now. Your health is more important than the few cents they cost. If your store doesn't carry these types of oils, check the resources in the back of this book.

The majority of vegetable oils today, even many health food store brands, are highly processed and refined. In the refining process, the oil is separated from its source with petroleum solvents and then boiled to evaporate the solvents. The oil is refined, bleached, and deodorized, which involves heating to temperatures of about 400 degrees F. Chemical preservatives are frequently added to retard oxidation.

The less processing an oil undergoes, the less harmful it is. The most natural oils are extracted from seeds by mechanical pressure and low temperatures, and without the use of chemicals. Oils derived by this process are referred to as "expeller pressed" or "cold pressed." These are the only vegetable oils you should eat. But be careful; even these oils are subject to oxidation and must be packaged, stored, and used properly.

SATURATED FATS

One distinct advantage that all saturated fats have over unsaturated fats (mono- and polyunsaturated fats) is that they don't have any missing hydrogen atoms or double-bonded carbons. This means that they are not vulnerable to oxidation and free-radical formation as unsaturated fats are. Food manufacturers have known this for decades. They've added saturated fats (often coconut and palm kernel oils) to foods because they help prevent spoilage caused by free radicals.

Over the years the tropical oils have been replaced in most foods by hydrogenated and partially hydrogenated oils. Hydrogenation is a process where an unsaturated vegetable oil is chemically altered to form a more saturated fat. Increasing the saturation makes the oil less susceptible to spoilage and is cheaper than using animal or tropical oils. Hydrogenation involves heating oils to high temperatures while bombarding them with hydrogen atoms, thus creating toxic trans fatty acids. These artificial fats are structurally different from natural fats. Our bodies can handle natural fats, but trans fatty acids have no place in our bodies and are linked to many health problems. Shortening and margarine are two hydrogenated oils that should be completely eliminated from your diet.

In the 1950s and 1960s, when saturated fat was first being associated with elevated cholesterol, researchers began looking for other potentially adverse effects caused by saturated fat. They reasoned that if excessive consumption of saturated fat increased the risk of developing heart disease, it might be associated with other health problems as well. Researchers began studying the relationship between saturated fat and cancer. What they found surprised them. When compared with other oils, it appeared that saturated fat had a *protective* effect against cancer rather than a causative one. Processed nonhydrogenated polyunsaturated oils were identified as promoting cancer, and the higher the degree of unsaturation, the greater the risk.

Other conditions such as asthma, allergies, memory loss, and senility also showed a greater degree of occurrence among people who use refined polyunsaturated oils rather than saturated fats. Another problem with these polyunsaturated oils is their influence on the immune system. Our immune system is what keeps us healthy. Polyunsaturated oils suppress the immune system, making us more vulnerable to disease and premature aging. Unsaturated fats not only suppress the immune system but can even kill white blood cells. The health of your immune system in large part determines your ability to ward off disease and remain healthy. Researchers believe that for the most part, free radicals are to blame for these conditions. When you eat conventionally processed polyunsaturated oils, the type typically sold in grocery stores, you are just shortening your life by providing a doorway for disease.

Because saturated fats have no double-carbon bonds—the weak links that are easily broken to form free radicals—they are much more stable under a variety of conditions. They can be exposed to heat, light, and oxygen without undergoing any appreciable degree of oxidation or free-radical formation. For this reason, they are preferable for use with food, especially if the food is going to be cooked or stored for any length of time. Saturated fat remains stable even when heated to normal cooking temperatures. This is why it is far superior to polyunsaturated oil for cooking purposes.

Coconut oil, being a highly saturated fat, is the least vulnerable of all the dietary oils to oxidation and free-radical formation and therefore is the safest to use in cooking. In addition, since it is composed primarily of medium-chain fatty acids, it is not like the long-chain saturated fatty acids that raise blood cholesterol levels. And unlike almost all saturated and unsaturated oils, it does not promote the platelet stickiness that leads to blood clot formation. Compared to other oils, coconut oil is rather benign, causing no harm. Replacing the liquid vegetable oils you are now using with coconut oil can help eliminate the many health problems caused by consuming oxidized oils. While coconut oil's apparent harmlessness is a definite advantage, it is not the primary reason it is so good. The medium-chain fatty acids in coconut oil give it properties that make it unique and considered by many to be the healthiest oil on earth.

TRANS FATTY ACIDS

Trans fatty acids are created by modern technology and are foreign to the human body. Because these fats are unlike the natural fatty acids needed for good health, our bodies are incapable of utilizing them in a productive manner. It's like pouring apple cider into the gas tank of your car—it gums up the works. Cars are designed to run on gasoline, not apple cider. The sugars in the apple juice will cause the engine to freeze up. In like manner, trans fatty acids cause our cells to freeze up, so to speak, leaving them dysfunctional. The more trans fatty acids eaten, the greater the cellular destruction, until entire tissues and organs become seriously affected. Disease is the result.

In the extraction, refining, and deodorizing process, vegetable oils are heated to temperatures up to 400 degrees F for extended periods of time. Vegetable oils are often hydrogenated to turn them into solid fats. In the process of hydrogenation, higher temperatures and longer exposure times create a far greater number of trans fatty acids. Shortening and margarine are hydrogenated oils. On average they contain about 35 percent trans fatty acids, but some brands may run as high as 48 percent. Between 15 and 19 percent of the fatty acids in conventionally processed liquid vegetable oils are trans fatty acids.

Many researchers believe trans fatty acids have a greater influence on the development of cardiovascular disease than any other dietary fat. Studies now clearly show that trans fatty acids can contribute to atherosclerosis and heart disease. For example, in animal studies, swine fed a diet containing trans fatty acids developed more extensive atherosclerotic damage than those fed other types of fats.

Researchers estimate that in the United States consumption of trans fatty acids causes at least 30,000 premature deaths a year! The *New England Journal of Medicine* reported the results of a 14-year study of more than 80,000 nurses (*New England Journal of Medicine,* November 20, 1997). The research documented 939 heart attacks among the participants. Among the women who consumed the largest amounts of trans fats, the chance of suffering a heart attack was 53 percent higher than that among those at the low end of trans fat consumption. Another interesting fact uncovered by this study was that total fat intake had little effect on the rate of heart attack. Women in the group with the largest consumption of total fat (46 percent of calories) had no greater risk of heart attack than those in the group with the lowest consumption of total fat (29 percent of calories).

The researchers from the Harvard School of Public Health and Brigham and Women's Hospital in Boston who conducted the study said this suggested that limiting consumption of trans fats would be more effective in avoiding heart attacks than reducing overall fat intake. About 15 percent of the fat in the typical Western diet is trans fat.

Trans fatty acids affect more than just our cardiovascular health. According to Mary Enig, Ph.D., when monkeys were fed trans fat–containing margarine in their diets, their red blood cells did not bind insulin as well as when they were not fed trans fats, suggesting a relationship with diabetes. Trans fatty acids have been linked with a variety of adverse health effects, including cancer, heart disease, multiple sclerosis (MS), diverticulitis, complications of diabetes, and other degenerative conditions.

Hydrogenated oil is a product of technology and may be the most destructive food additive currently in common use. If you eat margarine, shortening, or hydrogenated or partially hydrogenated oils (common food additives), then you are consuming trans fatty acids. Many of the foods you buy in the store and in restaurants are prepared with or cooked in hydrogenated oil. Fried foods sold in grocery stores and restaurants are usually cooked in hydrogenated oil. Many frozen, processed foods are cooked or prepared in hydrogenated oils. Hydrogenated oils are used in making french fries, biscuits, cookies, crackers, chips, frozen pies, pizzas, peanut butter, cake frosting, candy, and ice cream substitutes such as mellorine.

The processed vegetable oils you buy in the store aren't much better. The heat used in the extraction and refining process also creates trans fatty acids. So that bottle of corn or safflower oil you have on the kitchen shelf contains some trans fatty acids even though it has not been hydrogenated. Unless the vegetable oil has been "cold pressed" or "expeller pressed," it contains trans fatty acids. Most of the common brands of vegetable oil and salad dressing contain trans fatty acids.

Saturated fats from any source are much more tolerant of the temperatures used in cooking and do not form trans fatty acids or create harmful free radicals; therefore, they make much better cooking oils. Saturated fats are the only fats that are safe to heat and cook with. Many people, however, are hesitant to use saturated fat because of concern about heart disease. But coconut oil is heart healthy and can be used in cooking without fear. It not only is resistant to heat but is an excellent oil for improving overall health.

MCT OILS

Medium-chain triglyceride oils (sometimes referred to as fractionated coconut oil) have become increasingly popular in sports nutrition and in intravenous formulas used in hospitals. You are likely to encounter this term in foods and supplements sold at health stores if you haven't already.

As you learned at the beginning of this chapter, fatty acids are usually packaged in groups of three. These packages are called triglycerides. Medium-chain triglyceride (MCT) oils are simply oils composed of 100 percent medium-chain fatty acids (MCFAs). These fatty acids are derived from coconut or palm kernel oils. Since the medium-chain fatty acids are associated with many health benefits, manufacturers have developed oils composed entirely of them. Coconut oil, in comparison, contains only 64 percent MCFA.

Some of the unique health benefits of the medium-chain fatty acids found in coconut oil have been known and enjoyed since the 1950s. Because of this, coconut and MCT oils have been and still are used in hospitals to treat malabsorption syndrome, cystic fibrosis, and epilepsy and to improve protein and fat metabolism and mineral absorption. Because of their superior nutritional benefits, MCFAs are used in hospital formulas to nourish seriously burned or critically ill patients. Coconut oil, and more recently MCT oil, has been an important ingredient in commercial baby formulas and is essential in hospital formulas for treating and nourishing premature infants. Athletes use MCFAs to reduce and control weight and increase exercise performance. You may also see MCT or fractionated coconut oil sold by itself for use as a dietary supplement or cooking oil.

The health benefits of MCFAs in coconut oil are many. Each of the individual MCFAs exert somewhat different yet complementary effects on the body, and all are important. The MCFAs in coconut oil are lauric acid (48 percent), caprylic acid (8 percent), and capric acid (7 percent), in addition to other beneficial fatty acids. Unlike coconut oil, MCT oil consists almost entirely of just two fatty acids; this oil is approximately 75 percent caprylic acid and 25 percent capric acid. In my opinion, this is a major drawback because it contains little or no lauric acid, which is probably the most important MCFA. As I will show in chapter 4, lauric acid is an extremely important nutrient that provides some very valuable health benefits. Coconut oil, rich in lauric acid, contains a complete set of MCFAs as well as other nutrients. It provides a balance of several fatty acids rather than just two and, unlike MCT, is completely natural. The fatty acids in MCT oil are extracted and purified from coconut oil, making it a manufactured rather than a natural oil.

The soap and cosmetic industry use lauric acid in the manufacture of cleansing agents. This leaves behind capric and caprylic acids as byproducts that can be cheaply used for other purposes. While not used in the cosmetic industry, these medium-chain fatty acids have important nutritional and pharmaceutical applications. They are used in a variety of supplements and dietary formulas, and they compose the bases of MCT oil.

3

A NEW WEAPON AGAINST HEART DISEASE

While having dinner with friends some time ago, I happened to mention that coconut oil was the healthiest oil one could use. A member of the group objected to my statement and responded emphatically, "Coconut oil is unhealthy; it causes heart disease." My rebuke was quick and simple, "That must be why all the Pacific Islanders died off hundreds of years ago." My antagonist didn't know how to respond to this statement. The simple fact is: Pacific Islanders, who live on traditional diets rich in coconut, don't get heart disease.

Coconuts have been a staple in the diets of Pacific Islanders for thousands of years. They eat them by the pound every day. Common sense would tell you that if they were as harmful as we are led to believe, all the islanders should have died off years ago. But until their adoption of modern foods, heart disease and other degenerative conditions were unheard of. Heart disease only appeared in island populations after traditional foods consisting of coconuts and coconut oil were replaced by modern processed foods and refined vegetable oils.

The early explorers who visited the South Sea islands in the sixteenth and seventeenth centuries described the islanders as being exceedingly strong, vigorously built, beautiful in body, and kindly disposed. The islanders gained a reputation for their beauty, excellent physical development, and good health. Some of the islands were viewed as the equivalent to the Garden of Eden where the inhabitants were near perfect in stature and appearance. Such observations may have even fueled interest in the folklore of a fountain of youth. Tales of a mystical island containing such a fountain had been popular for centuries in Europe and led explorers, such as Juan Ponce de Leon, to search in vain for the mythical waters. While a fountain whose waters brought eternal youth was not to be found, the islanders did have a fountain of youth of sorts. That fountain was in the fruit of the coconut tree, the Tree of Life, as they call it. The coconut, with its life-giving water (the oil and milk), bestowed a level of youthful health on these people that far surpassed that of their European visitors.

It wasn't until relatively recently that science began to unlock the secrets to the islanders' good health and discover the many healing miracles of coconut oil. Through the pioneering research of people like Weston A. Price, Ian A. Prior, Jon J. Kabara, and others, we now know that it was the coconut-based diet that was largely responsible for the Islanders' good health and youthful appearance. It was and still is the reason Pacific Islanders don't get heart disease.

THE PUKAPUKA AND TOKELAU STUDIES

It has long been observed that people of the Pacific Islands and Asia, whose diets are high in coconut, are surprisingly free from cardiovascular disease, cancer, and other degenerative diseases. Some of the most thorough research conducted on people who have a high-fat diet derived primarily from coconuts is the Pukapuka and Tokelau Island study. This was a long-term multidisciplinary study set up to evaluate the health of those living on island atolls and the consequences of migrating to New Zealand, where they are exposed to Western foods and influences. The Tokelau and Pukapuka studies were begun in the early 1960s and included the entire populations of both islands, which was about 2,500 people.

The islands of Pukapuka and Tokelau lie near the equator in the South Pacific. Pukapuka is an atoll in the Northern Cooks Islands, and Tokelau, another atoll, lies about 400 miles southeast. Both are under the jurisdiction of New Zealand. The populations of both islands have been relatively isolated from Western influences. Their native diet and culture remain much as they have for centuries. Pukapuka and Tokelau are among the more isolated Polynesian islands and have had relatively little interaction with non-Polynesians.

The coral sands of these atolls are porous, lack humus, and will not support the food plants that flourish on other tropical islands. Coconut palms and a few starchy tropical fruits and root vegetables supply the vast majority of the diet for the population. Fish from the ocean, pigs, and chickens make up what little meat they eat. Some flour, rice, sugar, and canned meat are obtained from small cargo ships that occasionally visit the islands. Their diet is high in fiber but low in sugar.

The standard diet on both islands is high in fat derived from coconuts but remains low in cholesterol. Every meal contains coconut in some form: the green nut provides the main beverage; the mature nut, grated or as coconut cream, is cooked with taro root, breadfruit, or rice; and small pieces of coconut meat make an important snack food. Plants and fruitfish are cooked with coconut oil. In Tokelau, coconut sap or toddy is used as a sweetener and as leavening for bread.

The researchers reported that the overall health of both groups was extremely good compared to Western standards. There were no signs of kidney disease or hypothyroidism that might influence fat levels, and no hypercholesterolemia (high blood cholesterol). All inhabitants were lean and healthy, despite a very high-saturated-fat diet. In fact, the populations as a whole had ideal weight-to-height ratios as compared to the Body Mass Index figures used by nutritionists. Digestive problems were rare, constipation uncommon. The people averaged two or more bowel movements a day. Atherosclerosis, heart disease, colitis, colon cancer, hemorrhoids, ulcers, diverticulosis, and appendicitis are conditions with which they were generally unfamiliar.

SATURATED-FAT CONSUMPTION

The American Heart Association recommends that we get no more than 30 percent of our total calories from fat and that saturated fat should be limited to no more than 10 percent, but the Tokelauans apparently aren't aware of these guidelines—nearly 60 percent of their energy is derived from fat, and almost all of that is saturated fat derived largely from coconuts. The fat in the Pukapukan diet is also primarily from saturated fatty acids from coconut, with total energy from fat at 35 percent.

Most Americans and others who eat typical Western diets get 32–38 percent of their calories from fat, most of which is in the form of unsaturated vegetable oils. Yet they still suffer from numerous degenerative conditions and weight problems. In contrast, the islanders in this study consumed as much or more total fat and a far greater amount of saturated fat than typical Americans yet were relatively free from degenerative disease and generally lean and healthy.

Dr. Ian A. Prior and his colleagues calculated the cholesterol levels of the islanders based on rates observed in Western countries. The islanders' actual blood cholesterol levels were 70 to 80 milligrams lower than predicted, ranging from about 170 to 208 milligrams per deciliter. Cholesterol levels of the Tokelauans were the higher of the two because they derived 57 percent of total calories from fat, about 50 percent from saturated fat. Their total food consumption, including imported flour, rice, sugar, and meat, was also higher. Dietary cholesterol and polyunsaturated fatty acids of both groups were low. Dr. Prior noted that vascular disease is uncommon in both populations, and there is no evidence that the high–saturated-fat intake from coconut has a harmful effect.

DIETARY CHANGES
AFFECT HEALTH STATUS

The migration of Tokelau Islanders from their island atolls to the very different environment of New Zealand was associated with changes in fat intake that indicate increased risk of atherosclerosis. The migration was also associated with an actual decrease in saturated fat intake from about 50 percent to 41 percent of energy, an increase in dietary cholesterol intake to 340 milligrams, and an increase in polyunsaturated fat and sugar. Fat changes included increased total cholesterol, higher LDL (bad cholesterol) and triglycerides, and lower HDL (good cholesterol) levels.

The blood cholesterol of Tokelau Islanders increased when they migrated to New Zealand, despite the fact that the total fat content of their diet dropped, declining from 57 percent in Tokelau, with 80 percent of that from coconut oil, to around 43 percent in New Zealand. They ate more white bread, rice, meat, and other Western foods and less of their high-fiber, coconut-rich foods.

The conclusion we can make from these island studies is that a high-saturated-fat diet consisting of coconut oil is not detrimental to health and does not contribute to arteriosclerosis. Indeed, those people who eat coconut oil in place of other vegetable oils are amazingly free from the degenerative diseases that are so common in the West. They also have nearly ideal body weight and appear to be examples of perfect health. But when these people replace coconut oil in their diets with other oils and processed foods (which are typically loaded with polyunsaturated and hydrogenated oils) their health declines.

SATURATED FAT AND CHOLESTEROL

Saturated fat has been labeled a dietary villain that should be avoided at all costs. We buy lean cuts of meat, nonfat milk, and low-fat foods of all types in order to limit our intake of this dreaded substance. But why is saturated fat so bad? There is really only one suggested reason: saturated fat is easily converted by the liver into cholesterol, which can raise blood cholesterol levels, increasing the risk of heart disease.

But, contrary to popular belief, neither saturated fat nor cholesterol *cause* heart disease. This is a fact that all fat researchers and medical professionals know but many of the rest of us do not. High blood cholesterol is only one of many so-called risk factors associated with heart disease. What this means is that those people who have heart disease sometimes also have elevated blood cholesterol levels. Not all people with high blood cholesterol develop heart disease, and not everyone with heart disease has high blood cholesterol. If high blood cholesterol were the cause of heart disease, everybody who dies from this disease would have elevated cholesterol levels, but they don't. In fact, most people who have heart disease do not have high blood cholesterol.

Other risk factors associated with heart disease include high blood pressure, age, gender (being male), tobacco use, diabetes, obesity, stress, lack of exercise, insulin levels, and homocysteine levels. High blood cholesterol is no more the cause of heart disease than age or male gender is. It's guilty only by association.

Blood level of homocysteine is one of the most accurate of the risk factors. Recent research has shown that elevated homocysteine levels in the blood are much more strongly associated with heart disease than cholesterol. Homocysteine is an amino acid derived from protein found in meat, milk, and other foods. Homocysteine may help raise blood cholesterol, and the association of high blood cholesterol with heart disease may result more from homocysteine (derived primarily from protein found in meat and dairy products) than from cholesterol (or saturated fat).

The term "artery-clogging saturated fat" is a misnomer. The fat that collects in arterial plaque is primarily unsaturated fats (74 percent) and cholesterol. Saturated fat does not collect in the arteries like poly- and monounsaturated fats because it is not easily oxidized, and only oxidized fat ends up as arterial plaque. Vegetables oils are easily oxidized by over-processing and heating. Furthermore, saturated fat is not the only substance that your liver converts into cholesterol. Other fats, and even carbohydrate, the main nutritional component of all fruits, vegetables, and grains, also end up as cholesterol in our bodies. To infer that only saturated fat raises blood cholesterol is grossly inaccurate and misleading.

COCONUT OIL AND CHOLESTEROL

All of the criticism that has been aimed at coconut oil is based primarily on the fact that it is a saturated fat and saturated fat is known to increase blood cholesterol. No legitimate research, however, has ever demonstrated any proof that natural, nonhydrogenated coconut oil adversely affects blood cholesterol levels. In fact, numerous studies have clearly demonstrated that coconut oil has a neutral effect on cholesterol levels.

The reason coconut oil does not adversely affect cholesterol is because it is composed primarily of medium-chain fatty acids. These fatty acids are different from those commonly found in other food sources and are burned almost immediately for energy production, and so they are not converted into body fat or cholesterol to the degree other fats are and do not affect blood cholesterol levels.

While coconut oil's direct effect on blood cholesterol has generally been shown to be neutral, it may indirectly lower LDL (bad) cholesterol and increase HDL (good) cholesterol by stimulating metabolism (see chapter 5 for a more complete discussion on metabolic effects). In one study performed in the Philippines, for example, 10 medical students tested diets consisting of different levels of animal fat and coconut oil. Animal fat is known to raise blood cholesterol. Total calories from dietary fat consisted of 20 percent, 30 percent, and 40 percent, using different combinations of coconut oil and animal fat. At all three levels with a ratio of 1 to 1, 1 to 2, and 1 to 3, animal fat to coconut oil, no significant change in cholesterol levels was observed. Only when the ratio was reversed so that animal fat consumption was greater than coconut oil and when total fat calories reached 40 percent was a significant increase in blood cholesterol reported. This study demonstrated that not only did coconut oil not have a bad effect on cholesterol levels, it even reduced the cholesterol-elevating effects of animal fat.

CLOTTING AND HEART DISEASE

One of the important factors that influences cardiovascular health is the blood's tendency to form clots. When you cut yourself, proteins in your blood called platelets stick together and form a clot, which prevents your bleeding to death. In healthy people, the blood becomes sticky only when it comes in contact with a wound or injury. But when platelets stick to arterial walls, they can form dangerous clots that can block the flow of blood and cause a heart attack or stroke. In recent heart attack victims, the blood in their bodies has been found to be about 4.5 times stickier than that in normal people.

As a result, many doctors warn against saturated fat, as it has been blamed for increasing platelet adhesiveness (blood stickiness), thus promoting the development of blood clots. Some of the long-chain saturated fats, like those found in beef fat, lard, and butter, do increase platelet stickiness. But what is often left unsaid is that most polyunsaturated fats found in vegetable oils also promote clotting. In fact, all dietary oils, both saturated and unsaturated, with the exception of the omega-3 fatty acids (e.g., flaxseed oil, fish oil) and the medium-chain fatty acids (e.g., tropical oils), increase platelet stickiness. Even the so-called heart-healthy olive oil increases blood clot risk. So when you eat corn, safflower, soybean, cottonseed, canola, and peanut oils you are increasing your risk of suffering a heart attack or stroke. Eating omega-3 fatty acids and MCFAs, like coconut oil, has the opposite effect on blood platelets. Medium-chain fatty acids are burned up immediately after consumption and therefore do not affect platelet stickiness either one way or the other. Studies have revealed that populations who traditionally consume large quantities of coconut as a part of their diet have a low incidence of health problems associated with blood clotting, including heart disease and stroke.

ATHEROSCLEROSIS AND HEART DISEASE

To understand how coconut oil can help prevent heart disease, you need to have a basic understanding of how the disease develops. Heart disease is caused by atherosclerosis, or hardening of the arteries, which is manifested by the formation of plaque in the arteries. If you asked most people what causes atherosclerosis, they would probably tell you it was from too much cholesterol in the blood. But cholesterol doesn't simply come dancing freely down the artery and suddenly decide to stick somewhere. In fact, cholesterol isn't even necessary for atherosclerosis or the formation of plaque. The body uses cholesterol to patch up and repair injuries to the arterial wall. Contrary to popular belief, the principle component of arterial plaque is not cholesterol but protein, mainly in the form of scar tissue. Some atherosclerotic arteries actually contain little or no cholesterol.

According to the response-to-injury hypothesis, atherosclerosis initially develops as a result of injury to the inner lining of the arterial wall. The injury can be the result of a number of factors such as toxins, free radicals, viruses, or bacteria. If the cause of the injury is not removed, further damage may result, and as long as irritation and inflammation persist, scar tissue continues to develop.

When blood-clotting proteins (platelets) encounter an injury, they become sticky and adhere to each other and to the damaged tissue, acting somewhat like a bandage to facilitate healing. This is how blood clots are formed. Injury from any source triggers platelets to clump together, or clot, and arterial cells to release protein growth factors that stimulate growth of the muscle cells within the artery walls. A complex mixture of scar tissue, platelets, calcium, cholesterol, and triglycerides is incorporated into the site to heal the injury. This mass of fibrous tissue, not cholesterol, forms the principle material in plaque. The calcium deposits in the plaque cause the hardening, which is characteristic of atherosclerosis.

Contrary to popular belief, plaque isn't simply plastered along the inside of the artery canal like mud in a garden hose. It grows inside the artery wall, becoming part of the artery wall itself. Arterial walls are surrounded by a layer of strong circular muscles that prevent the plaque

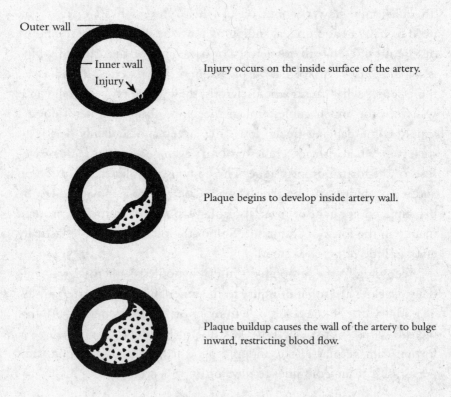

Outer wall

Inner wall
Injury

Injury occurs on the inside surface of the artery.

Plaque begins to develop inside artery wall.

Plaque buildup causes the wall of the artery to bulge inward, restricting blood flow.

from expanding outward. As the plaque grows, because it can't expand outward, it begins to push inward and close the artery opening, narrowing the artery and choking off blood flow.

Platelets gather at the site of injury to form blood clots, plugging the holes in the damaged vessel. But if the injury persists or if the blood is prone to clotting, clots may continue to grow to the point that they completely block the artery. An artery already narrowed by plaque can easily be blocked by blood clots. When this process occurs in the coronary artery, which feeds the heart, it is referred to as a heart attack. If it happens in the carotid artery, which goes to the brain, the result is a stroke.

CHRONIC INFECTION AND ATHEROSCLEROSIS

Although many risk factors are associated with heart disease, none has actually been proven to cause the illness. Lack of exercise is a risk factor just as high blood cholesterol is, but neither one actually causes heart disease. If lack of physical activity caused heart disease, then everyone who doesn't exercise would die of a heart attack, but they don't. Likewise, everyone with high cholesterol doesn't get heart disease, and everyone who has heart disease doesn't have high cholesterol. Risk is only an observed association and not necessarily a cause. A substantial proportion of people with heart disease, however, do not have any of the standard risk factors. The actual cause of heart disease is elusive and appears to be multifactorial.

One area of investigation that is gaining a great deal of interest is the relationship between chronic infection and atherosclerosis. It appears that there is a cause-and-effect relationship associated with persistent low-grade infections and heart disease. Recent research has shown that certain microorganisms can cause or are at least involved in the development of arterial plaque, which leads to heart disease.

A large number of studies have reported associations between heart disease and chronic bacterial and viral infections. As far back as the 1970s researchers identified the development of atherosclerosis in the arteries of chickens when they were experimentally infected with a herpes virus. In the 1980s similar associations were reported in humans infected with a number of bacteria (e.g., *Helicobacter pylori* and *Chlamydia pneumoniae*) and certain herpes viruses (particularly cytomegalovirus). In one study, for example, Petra Saikku and her colleagues at the University of Helsinki in Finland found that 27 out of 40 heart attack patients and 15 out of 30 men with heart disease carried antibodies related to chlamydia, which is more commonly known to cause gum disease and lung infections. In subjects who were free of heart disease, only 7 out of 41 had such antibodies. In another study at Baylor College of Medicine in Houston, Texas, researchers found that 70 percent of patients undergoing surgery for atherosclerosis carried antibodies to cytomegalovirus (CMV), a common respiratory infection, while only 43 percent of controls did.

More evidence supporting the link between infection and cardiovascular disease showed up in the early 1990s, when researchers found fragments of bacteria in arterial plaque. One of the first to discover microorganisms in atherosclerotic plaque was Brent Muhlestein, a cardiologist at the LDS Hospital in Salt Lake City and the University of Utah. Muhlestein and colleagues found evidence of chlamydia in 79 percent of plaque specimens taken from the coronary arteries of 90 heart disease patients. In comparison, fewer than 4 percent of normal individuals had evidence of chlamydia in artery walls. Animal studies provided more direct evidence that bacteria might contribute to chronic inflammation and plaque formation. Muhlestein showed that infecting rabbits with chlamydia measurably thickens the arterial walls of the animals. When the animals were given an antibiotic to kill the chlamydia, the arteries became more normal in size.

At least one out of every two adults in developed countries has antibodies to *Helicobacter pylori*, *Chlamydia pneumoniae*, or cytomegalovirus

(CMV). The presence of antibodies does not necessarily indicate an active infection or the presence of atherosclerosis, but it is a sign that infection has occurred at some time. It's common for infections from these organisms to persist indefinitely. Once one is infected with herpes, for example, the virus remains for life. The effectiveness of the immune system determines the degree of trouble the virus may cause. The weaker the immune system, the more likely an infection is to hang on and cause problems. When these microorganisms enter the bloodstream they can attack the artery wall, causing chronic low-grade infections that lack any noticeable symptoms. As microorganisms colonize an artery wall, they cause damage to arterial cells. In an effort to heal the injury, blood platelets, cholesterol, and protein combine in the artery wall, setting the stage for plaque formation and atherosclerosis. As long as the infection and inflammation persist, plaque continues to develop. Infection can both initiate and promote growth of atherosclerosis in arteries, which in turn, leads to heart disease.

At this point, researchers are not ready to say that infection is responsible for every case of heart disease. Other factors (e.g., free radicals, high blood pressure, diabetes, etc.) can also cause injuries to the arterial wall and initiate plaque formation. And not all infections promote atherosclerosis. Only when the immune system is incapable of controlling the infection is there cause for alarm. Anything that may lower immune efficiency, such as serious illness, poor diet, exposure to cigarette smoke, stress, and lack of exercise (i.e., many of the typical risk factors associated with heart disease), will also open up the body to chronic low-grade infections that can promote atherosclerosis.

We now know that, at least in some cases, heart disease may be treated with antibiotics. But antibiotics are limited because they work only against bacteria, and infections caused by viruses remain unaffected. However, there is something that will destroy both the bacteria (*Helicobacter pylori* and *Chlamydia pneumoniae*) and viruses (CMV) that are most commonly associated with atherosclerosis, and that is MCFAs, or coconut oil. Yes, believe it or not. The MCFAs in coconut oil are known to kill all three of the major types of atherogenic organisms. These special fatty acids are harmless to us and even provide us nourishment and energy but are deadly to microorganisms that cause infection and illness. Research has shown that MCFAs from coconut oil can kill bacteria and viruses that cause influenza, herpes, bladder infections, gum disease, and numerous other conditions. Coconut oil provides a safe and effective way to prevent and even overcome many common illnesses. This topic is discussed in more detail in the following chapter.

FREE-RADICAL INJURY

Another major cause of arterial injury that can lead to atherosclerosis is free radicals. These renegade molecules, found in tobacco smoke, polluted air, and many substances in our food and environment, can cause damage to cells and tissues wherever they are allowed to roam. Probably the dietary substances most dangerous to the heart and arteries are the oxidized lipids (fats) found in rancid fats and refined oils that have been stripped of natural antioxidants. Oxidized fats are abundant in our modern diet, especially in processed vegetable oils, and they have been found to accumulate in arterial plaque.

The only way to stop a free radical is with an antioxidant. Antioxidants are molecules that neutralize free radicals, making them harmless. Numerous studies have shown that diets high in fruits and vegetables rich in antioxidants (vitamins A, C, and E and beta-carotene) reduce the risk of heart disease and stroke. If antioxidants are readily available in the bloodstream, they can protect the arteries from free-radical injury and reduce risk of heart disease.

We can get antioxidants in fresh fruits and vegetables, but most people don't eat enough of these to provide significant protection. Antioxidant supplements can help, and so can coconut oil. Unlike other vegetable oils, coconut oil is chemically very stable and is not oxidized easily. In fact, it is so resistant to free-radical attack that it acts as an antioxidant, helping to prevent the oxidation of other oils. Coconut oil protects the heart and arteries from injury caused by bacteria, viruses, and free radicals. By removing the cause of arterial injury, coconut oil prevents further damage, allowing the arterial walls to heal, thus not only reducing risk of heart disease but actually promoting healing.

DENTAL HEALTH AND HEART DISEASE

A remarkable series of studies of the health of Pacific Island populations was conducted in the 1930s, when Dr. Weston A. Price, a dentist and nutritional researcher from Cleveland, Ohio, traveled to the islands to study the relationship between the islanders' health and their diet. His results were published in 1938 in a book titled *Nutrition and Physical Degeneration*. This book, which is still in print, is considered a classic in nutritional science.

His travels took him to numerous islands scattered over thousands of miles of the Pacific Ocean. He studied native populations in Hawaii, Samoa, Fiji, Tahiti, Raratonga, Nukualofa, New Caledonia, the Marquesas, and other islands. In the 1930s many of the people still lived as they had for generations, eating traditional foods. Commercial trade with the islanders brought Western foods and influences to the ports of many of these islands. As a result, many islanders had adopted the Western way of life, including its foods. This provided Dr. Price with an ideal setting for studying the differences between native and modern diets and how they each affect health.

Being a dentist, Dr. Price focused his research on dental health, but he also made note of health in general. He examined and analyzed the food and diets of the people. He immediately noticed the contrast in health between those who lived entirely on indigenous foods, such as coconut and taro root, and those who had abandoned their traditional diet for Western foods.

Wherever he found islanders living on traditional foods, he noted that both their dental and physical health were excellent, but when the islanders abandoned traditional foods and began eating modern foods, their health declined. In the absence of modern medical care, physical degeneration was pronounced. Dental disease, as well as infectious and degenerative diseases such as arthritis and tuberculosis, became common. For instance, the New Caledonian islanders who lived near the ports where modern foods were available had an incidence of dental caries (cavities) of 26 percent, and those who lived inland and on a diet of native foods an incidence of 0.14 percent. Those who lived near the ports also had a higher instance of gum disease and other health problems.

This wasn't an isolated phenomenon seen on only one or two islands. The same pattern repeated itself over and over again. In fact, every population he studied displayed this pattern. He found no exceptions. Overall, Dr. Price found that the number of teeth affected by cavities among those who ate traditional native foods was only about 0.3 percent (3 out of every 1,000 teeth examined) while the number of cavities in westernized islanders was typically as much as 30 percent (3 out of 10). He noted, as do many dentists nowadays, that the health of the mouth reflects the overall health of the individual. People with poor dental health also suffer from many other health problems; people who have good dental health are generally very healthy overall. Recent studies have verified this observation. Some of the conditions associated with dental disease include: heart disease, stroke, atherosclerosis, diabetes, ulcers, and pneumonia.

In all these island populations, coconut, in one form or another, was a staple part of the diet; for some it was their primary source of food. The amount of fat (primarily from coconuts) in their diet far exceeded that in those in the West, yet both their dental and overall health was far superior. Through Dr. Price's studies we see that eating coconuts and coconut oil didn't harm the islanders one bit. If anything, it gave them a higher level of health than most of us.

DENTAL HEALTH—A KEY TO UNDERSTANDING HEART DISEASE

A wise farmer, when considering buying a horse, always examines its mouth. He knows that the condition of the animal's mouth reflects the health of its entire body. No farmer in his right mind is going to pay top dollar for an animal with missing teeth or sore gums. Dental problems signal that other health problems are likely to be present. This is true with humans as well. This fact was recognized long ago and was the basis for the old focal-infection theory used in dentistry. According to this theory, an oral infection can influence the health of the whole body. On the basis of this theory, old-time dentists were inclined to pull all diseased teeth in the hope of preventing disease from spreading to other parts of the body. In the mid–twentieth century, better dental techniques were developed, teeth were repaired without being pulled, and the focal-infection theory came to be ignored. Fixing the teeth, however, doesn't stop the association between dental disease and health. People can have good-looking teeth but still have recurring episodes of dental disease as well as other health problems. In recent years the focal-infection theory has made a comeback. Poor oral health has been linked with numerous health problems, including diabetes and ulcers, but the most striking correlation is with cardiovascular illnesses such as heart disease, stroke, and atherosclerosis.

Several studies have found that heart disease patients have more tooth decay and higher rates of gum disease. The reverse is also true. Those with poor dental health are more likely to suffer a heart attack. Subjects in these studies had their dental health evaluated and then were monitored for several years to see if those with poor dental health were more likely to get heart disease. They were. For example, Robert J. Genco, D.D.S., Ph.D., of the University of Buffalo, studied 1,372 people over a 10-year period and found that heart disease was three times more prevalent for those with gum disease. In the National Health and Nutritional Examination Study published in the *British Medical Journal* (vol. 306, pp. 688–91) people with inflammation of the gums had a 25 percent increased risk of heart disease. Risk was high even for those who had gum disease in the past as well as currently. From these studies it appears that those who have or have had dental infections have a much higher risk of developing heart disease.

Some researchers believe that oral bacteria that cause dental disease enter the bloodstream through small tears in the gums. In the circulatory system these bacteria can cause inflammation, increase blood clotting, and promote the formation of arterial plaque, all of which leads to heart disease, as well as stroke and atherosclerosis.

Others have proposed that the bacteria responsible for heart and gum disease are present in the body because of poor diet and lifestyle choices that weaken the body's natural defenses. To some extent these bacteria are present in the body all the time, but if the body is strong and healthy, the bacteria do not reach numbers that would cause problems. In this view, gum disease does not necessarily lead to heart disease; they each happen at the same time, more or less, as a result of the body's inability to adequately control the bacteria.

It seems that if you have good dental health you are likely to have good cardiovascular health as well. This is interesting because the Pacific Islanders that Dr. Price studied never brushed their teeth, never flossed, never used antibacterial mouthwash, and never saw dentists; yet they had exquisite dental health, that is, as long as they continued to eat their traditional, coconut-based diet. The islanders' good dental health was a reflection of the absence of heart disease and other degenerative conditions.

MONEY, POLITICS, AND HEART DISEASE

Unlike the standard treatments for heart disease, coconut oil is cheap, has no adverse side effects, and is readily available to everyone. This, however, may also be a drawback. Because it is a natural product that is already widely available, pharmaceutical and medical industries have no desire to fund studies or promote interest in this area. There is no profit for them. Since most of the information on MCFAs and coconut oil are buried in scientific literature, few people are aware of the benefits. Knowledge about the true health aspects of coconut oil has to come from experienced clinicians, authors, and researchers who are familiar with the true facts about coconut oil. Yet they face an uphill battle because they must fight prejudice and misguided popular opinion that is fueled by powerful profit-seeking enterprises.

The soybean industry's attack on tropical oils was built on the accusation that these oils cause heart disease. This is ironic because replacing tropical oils with hydrogenated vegetable oils has actually increased heart disease deaths. And they know it. As far back as the 1950s, hydrogenated oils were suspected of causing heart disease. The soybean industry, fully aware that hydrogenated oils caused health problems, attempted to discourage and even suppress studies that presented unfavorable results. In the book *What Your Doctor Won't Tell You,* Jane Heimlich tells about one researcher who, after publishing the results of a study unfavorable to hydrogenated oils, found that she could no longer find funding. The purpose of her research, she thought, was to reveal truth and increase knowledge, not promote a product, but this didn't set well with the vegetable oil industry, and they refused to fund any of her future studies.

The truth about hydrogenated oils and trans fatty acids eventually emerged. Like the tobacco industry, which denied for years that cigarette smoke caused cancer, the soybean industry has denied that trans fatty acids promote heart disease. They cunningly diverted the public's attention to saturated fats and tropical oils, pointing a finger and calling them the troublemakers. In the 1980s and early 1990s, as the soybean industry's campaign against tropical oils raged, study after study implicated hydrogenated oils in contributing to heart disease as well as to a number of other health problems. Aware of the growing evidence against hydrogenated oils, the soybean industry conveniently avoided discussing this in their anti–tropical oil campaign. They always implied that tropical oils should be replaced by "vegetable oils." They didn't say what type of vegetable oil, but they knew all along that it would be hydrogenated vegetable oil.

As knowledge of the benefits of coconut oil increases, the soybean industry and its friends will step up their efforts to confuse the public with unfounded criticism and research funding designed to hide the truth and to make its products appear more desirable. Biased research in favor of the funding institution or industry happens all too often. Smear campaigns like those sponsored in the 1980s and early 1990s will undoubtedly continue.

A NEW LOOK AT COCONUT OIL

One of the biggest tragedies of our time concerning diet and health is the mistaken belief that coconut oil is a dietary villain that causes heart disease. Ironically, it may be one of best things you can eat to help protect you from heart disease. Instead of being a villain, as it is often made out to be, it is in reality a saint. By eating coconut oil you can reduce your chances of suffering a heart attack!

As I have shown, coconut oil does not increase blood cholesterol levels, nor does it promote platelet stickiness (excessive blood-clot formation). Because it stimulates metabolism it may, in fact, promote lower cholesterol. Studies in the 1970s and 1980s indicated that coconut oil is heart friendly, even though saturated fat at the time was being accused of promoting heart disease. Coconut oil consumption was found to have many factors associated with a reduced risk of heart disease, compared to those of other dietary oils, namely, lower body-fat deposition, higher survival rate, reduced tendency to form blood clots, fewer uncontrolled free radicals in cells, lower levels of blood and liver cholesterol, higher antioxidant reserves in cells, and lower incidence of heart disease in population studies.

Coconut oil also seems to have a direct effect on the heart itself. In my practice, I have seen it help regulate heart function and lower blood pressure. For example, Maria, a heart disease patient, was told by her cardiologist that she had only five years to live. One of the common symptoms of heart disease is cardiac arrhythmia—an accelerated, irregular heartbeat. She suffered so severely from arrhythmia that her doctor insisted she have a pacemaker implanted in her chest. She refused. She tried many natural methods, but her symptoms persisted and worsened. I told her about coconut oil, and she began taking it like a dietary supplement—4 tablespoons a day. The very first day she reported that her arrhythmia had decreased by about 50 percent. She reported that it was the calmest her heart had been in years. Nothing she had ever tried before had worked this well. She continues to take coconut oil, and her heart is functioning more normally now. While I was overjoyed to hear of Maria's success, it really wasn't a surprise. People who are familiar with coconut have learned that it helps the heart. As they say in Jamaica, "Coconut is a health tonic, good for the heart."

Heart disease, stroke, and atherosclerosis account for nearly half of all the deaths in most developed countries. Statistically, nearly one out of every two people you know will die from one of these cardiovascular conditions. In contrast, those people throughout the world who eat the most coconut have the lowest rates of heart disease in the world. For example, up until a few years ago the people of Sri Lanka used coconut oil in all their cooking. Each person consumed the equivalent of 120 coconuts a year. Despite their large coconut oil consumption heart disease is relatively rare. Only one out of every 100,000 deaths was due to heart disease.

In the coconut-growing regions of India the people were told to stop eating coconut oil because it caused heart disease. They began eating margarine and processed vegetable oils in place of coconut oil and within just a few years the heart disease rates tripled! Obviously coconut oil consumption did not cause the rise in heart disease. Researchers in India are now recommending the return to coconut oil to *reduce* the risk of heart disease.

From this evidence alone, coconut oil should be viewed as heart healthy, or at least benign, as far as heart disease is concerned. Coconut oil, however, is not simply a benign bystander but a very important player in the battle against heart disease. The evidence is so remarkable that coconut oil may soon become a powerful new weapon in the fight against heart disease.

4

NATURE'S MARVELOUS
GERM FIGHTER

There's nothing else we can do," the doctor said as the 57-year-old kidney patient lay dying. For nine months Dr. Gibert had desperately tried one antibiotic after another, but nothing worked. The man's blood remained flooded with bacteria, slowly poisoning his body.

"We tried six or seven different medications. Some we didn't think would work. But we had nothing else to try," said Gibert, an infectious disease specialist at the Veterans Affairs Medical Center in Washington, D.C. Even experimental drugs proved useless. Sometimes the man's blood tested clean, but within days the infection came roaring back. One strain of bacteria would die, but a few antibiotic-resistant bacteria would take the place of their more vulnerable cousins. Then they multiplied by the billions. The patient sensed his doctor's frustration.

"I guess you're going to tell me I'm dying," he sighed discouragingly.

"Nothing is working," she confided. "There are no more options."

Antibiotics, the miracle drugs of the twentieth century, had been useless against this new strain of bacteria, and within days the man died of a massive bacterial infection of the blood and heart.

Today people are suffering and dying from illnesses that science predicted 40 years ago would be wiped off the face of the earth. Infectious illnesses like tuberculosis, pneumonia, and sexually transmitted diseases, which were thought to have been conquered through the use of anti-biotics, have made a frightening comeback. Infectious diseases are now the third leading killer of Americans, after cancer and heart disease, and are becoming a global threat. "The world's population has never been more vulnerable to emerging and reemerging infections," wrote Dr. Joshua Lederberg, a Nobel Prize–winner for research in the genetic structure of microbes, in an editorial in the *Journal of the American Medical Association*.

Experts say our overuse of antibiotics is largely to blame: antibiotics encourage proliferation of drug-resistant bacteria. The Centers for Disease Control and Prevention (CDC) examined death records nation-wide and found 65 deaths among every 100,000 people were caused by infectious disease, up from 41 of every 100,000 deaths 12 years earlier. In 1946, just five years after penicillin came into wide use, doctors discovered a staphylococcus bacteria that was not vulnerable to the drug. Pharmacologists developed new antibiotics, but new drug-resistant bacteria appeared. As new drugs were developed, new strains of bacteria arose. By developing new drugs to combat the new strains of bacteria, pharmacologists thought they would be able to stay ahead. Slowly, scourges such as tuberculosis, bacterial pneumonia, septicemia (blood poisoning), syphilis, gonorrhea, and other bacterial infections were van-quished—or so it seemed. People still died from these ills, but not so many. In recent years, disease-causing bacteria have been staging a pow-erful comeback. We are in a new age of germ warfare—the age of the "supergerm."

Today every disease-causing bacterium has versions that resist at least one of medicine's 100-plus antibiotics. Some of these supergerms resist almost all known antibiotics. Drug-resistant tuberculosis now accounts for one in seven new cases. Several resistant strains of pneumococcus, the microbe responsible for infected surgical wounds and some chil-dren's ear infections and meningitis, appeared in the 1970s and are still going strong. Thousands of patients are now dying of bacterial infec-tions that were once cured by antibiotics. It isn't that their infections were immune to every single drug but rather that by the time doctors found an antibiotic that worked, the rampaging bacteria had poisoned the patient's blood or crippled some vital organ.

While medications are still an important defense against bacterial infections, the emergence of supergerms has increased our vulnerability to many diseases we thought would soon be rare or extinct. While antibiotics are losing ground to infectious organisms, nature has provided us an antibiotic that germs cannot develop a resistance to. That natural antibiotic is in the form of the MCFAs commonly found in coconut oil.

FOOD POISONING— A GROWING PROBLEM

Another growing concern in recent years is the sanitation practices in the food-processing industry. Food poisoning caused by bacteria is becoming a serious concern. Meat is the most common source of harmful bacteria. It easily becomes contaminated in slaughterhouses and warehouses, where sanitary conditions are often deplorable. Because of the prevalence of contamination in meat, we are continually advised to cook all meat thoroughly before eating. Even a tiny speck of blood on a cutting board or knife can transfer the bacteria to raw foods, leading to illness or even death.

The CDC estimate that in the United States up to three-quarters of all cases of food poisoning are directly linked to ground beef. A batch of ground beef might contain portions of meat from as many as 100 cows, any one of which may have been contaminated. It only takes a microscopic amount of meat from one infected animal to contaminate an entire batch of meat, and then this large batch of meat is divided and sent to dozens of stores and restaurants. The most notable outbreak occurred in 1993. Seven hundred people who ate Jack-in-the-Box hamburgers became ill, some sustaining permanent kidney damage, and at least four children died. *E. coli,* the culprit in the Jack-in-the-Box outbreak, kills an estimated 100 people a year in the United States and sickens 25,000 others.

Even foods we normally regard as safe can be a problem. For example, we think milk that has been pasteurized is free from harmful germs, but contamination can occur after pasteurization. In 1994 a truck that was contaminated with salmonella from a previous cargo of raw eggs delivered tainted pasteurized milk to an ice cream factory in Minnesota. The ice cream made from that milk was then shipped to stores in several states, causing an estimated 224,000 cases of food poisoning, the largest single food poisoning outbreak in U.S. history. Since then there have been over 50 major outbreaks in this country.

Between 6.5 million and 81 million Americans experience foodborne illnesses each year, and about 9,000 die as a result. While most cases don't end in death, food poisoning is far more common than we realize. Some experts estimate that as much as half of the flu cases that occur each year are actually reactions to food poisoning. The bout with the flu you experienced last fall may very well have really been food poisoning.

Contamination has become a growing problem not just with meat but with all types of food. Our fruits and vegetables aren't even safe. Unpasteurized apple cider, lettuce, and strawberries have also caused widespread outbreaks of food poisoning. While cooking destroys disease-causing bacteria, many fruits and vegetables are eaten raw. The only other thing you can do is wash your produce and hope you've cleaned it adequately enough. Then if you do become sick, antibiotics and your body's own recuperative powers are your only defense. But what if you're infected with one of the supergerms—say a strain of staphylococcus that is resistant to most antibiotics—what do you do? You'd better hope your immune system is strong enough to overcome it.

ALL VIRUSES ARE SUPERGERMS

Antibiotics still work for most bacterial infections; viruses, however, are another matter. They are all, in a sense, supergerms because there are no drugs that can effectively kill them. Antibiotics are only useful against bacteria, not viruses. To date, no drugs have been developed that can effectively eradicate viruses and cure the illnesses they cause. Antiviral drugs may reduce the severity of the infections but do not eliminate them completely. That is why there is no cure for the common cold—a viral infection. When you get a viral infection such as a cold, flu, herpes, or mononucleosis, there is little the doctor can do for you. The doctor's only option is to help you feel a little more comfortable by reducing the severity of the symptoms while your body fights the infection.

The most effective weapons against viruses are vaccines, but these are used to prevent disease, not treat it. Vaccines use dead or weakened viruses that are injected into the body. The body recognizes a vaccine as a viral infection and mounts a feverish attack by producing its own "anti-viral" compounds, called antibodies. These vaccines, however, have the potential to cause infections and other illnesses, so they aren't com-pletely safe. Viruses are continually mutating and new strains emerging, so vaccines for most of them aren't available. The only real protection against viral infections is our body's own natural defenses.

Because there is no cure for viral infections, they can become deadly, especially in individuals with depressed immunity. Many children and elderly die each year from flu that ordinarily would not be fatal. One of the most hideous outbreaks in modern times is AIDS, caused by the hu-man immunodeficiency virus (HIV). This virus attacks the cells of the immune system, leaving the person vulnerable to infection by any num-ber of opportunistic organisms. Infection by these organisms eventually causes the victim's death. As yet, none of the antiviral drugs can stop it.

When you catch a cold or get the flu, how long does it stay around? For most people it lasts several days to a week or more. There is no medicine, no cure, for the common cold or the flu. When you get sick, you have to let your body fight its own battle. That's why it takes so long to get rid of it.

Not too long ago an associate of mine said she felt like she was com-ing down with the flu. She had the beginnings of a sore throat, sinus congestion, and inklings of fatigue. I told her, "Take two to three ta-blespoons of coconut oil mixed in a glass of lukewarm orange juice with every meal." She looked at me inquisitively, as if to say "You've got to be joking. How is coconut oil going to help?"

From earlier discussions, she knew coconut oil had many nutritional benefits, but she doubted it would help with her infection. I didn't tell her it would cure her or that it would even make her feel any better. "Trust me," I said. "Take it and see what happens."

During the first day the symptoms got worse, as they usually do with seasonal infections. Normally, the flu gets progressively worse for the first few days until the body has had time to rally its defenses sufficiently to fight the invading infection. The next day, instead of getting worse, the symptoms started to go away. By the end of third day the symptoms were all but gone. Three days—that's all it took. She was surprised. "I never had an infection that lasted only three days," she said.

We are in the age of supergerms, and our environment is teaming with microorganisms. They are in the air we breathe, the food we eat, and the water we drink, and they even live on our skin. Many of these germs cause disease. Some have become drug-resistant supergerms. Fortunately, nature has provided us a number of medicinal plants to help protect us from attack by these harmful pests. Coconut is one of these. Medications can't be relied on to protect us against all infectious organisms. We need something more to boost our immune system and help us fight these troublesome invaders—a super antimicrobial.

COCONUT OIL: A SUPER ANTIMICROBIAL

When coconut oil is eaten, the body transforms its unique fatty acids into powerful antimicrobial powerhouses capable of defeating some of the most notorious disease-causing microorganisms. Even the supergerms are vulnerable to these lifesaving coconut derivatives. The unique properties of coconut oil make it, in essence, a natural antibacterial, antiviral, antifungal, and antiprotozoal food.

Fatty acids are essential to our health. We must have them in order to supply the building blocks for tissues and hormones. Every cell in our bodies must have a ready supply of fatty acids in order to function properly. Nature put fatty acids in our foods for a purpose. Your body recognizes them and knows what to do with them; MCFAs are natural substances the body knows how to use for its benefit. They are harmless to us while they are deadly to certain microorganisms.

Most bacteria and viruses are encased in a coat of lipids (fats). The fatty acids that make up this outer membrane or skin enclose the organism's DNA and other cellular materials. But, unlike our skin, which is relatively tough, the membrane of these microorganisms is nearly fluid. The fatty acids in the membrane are loosely attached, giving the membrane a remarkable degree of mobility and flexibility. This unique property allows these organisms to move, bend, and squeeze through the tiniest openings.

Lipid-coated viruses and bacteria are easily killed by MCFAs, which primarily destroy these organisms by disrupting their lipid membranes. Medium-chain fatty acids, being similar to those in the microorganism's membrane, are easily attracted to and absorbed into it. Unlike the other fatty acids in the membrane, MCFAs are much smaller and therefore weaken the already nearly fluid membrane to such a degree that it disintegrates. The membrane literally splits open, spilling its insides and killing the organism. Our white blood cells quickly clean up and dispose of the cellular debris. MCFAs kill invading organisms without causing any known harm to human tissues.

Our bodies have many ways of protecting us from harmful microorganisms. The strong acid excreted in our stomachs, for example, kills most of the organisms that we may eat with our foods. In our bloodstream, microorganisms are attacked and killed by our white blood cells. Our first line of defense against any harmful organism, however, is our skin. In order to inflict harm, microorganisms must first penetrate the skin's protective barrier. While the skin is permeable to some degree, it is also equipped with chemical weapons to help it ward off attack. One of these weapons is the oil secreted by our sebaceous (oil) glands. Sebaceous glands are found near the root of every hair. This oil is secreted along the hair shaft to lubricate the hair and skin. Some have described this oil as "nature's skin cream" because it prevents drying and cracking of the skin. It also has another very important function: It contains medium-chain fatty acids to fight invading microorganisms. A thin layer of oil on the skin helps protect us from the multitude of harmful germs our skin comes into contact with each day.

Besides being utilized on our skin to shield us from infectious intruders, MCFAs are found in mother's milk, to protect and nourish babies. They are nontoxic to us and create no toxic byproducts. They are completely safe and natural. The lipid researcher Jon J. Kabara, Ph.D., speaking of the safety of using fatty acids for medicinal purposes, says: "Fatty acids and derivatives tend to be the least toxic chemicals known to man. Not only are these agents nontoxic to man but [they] are actual foods and in the case of unsaturated fatty acids are essential to growth, development, and health."

While MCFAs, like caprylic acid and capric acid, demonstrate antimicrobial properties and have no undesirable or harmful side effects, lauric acid has the greatest antiviral activity. Coconut oil is composed of 48 percent lauric acid (a 12-chain saturated fatty acid), 7 percent capric acid (a 10-chain saturated fatty acid), 8 percent caprylic acid (an 8-chain saturated fatty acid), and 0.5 percent caproic acid (a 6-chain saturated fatty acid). These fatty acids give coconut oil its amazing antimicrobial properties and are generally absent from all other vegetable and animal oils, with the exception of butter.

LAURIC ACID

Technically speaking, coconut oil as it is found in fresh coconuts has little, if any, antimicrobial properties. Coconuts can be attacked by fungi and bacteria like any other fruit or nut. I know this sounds contrary to what I've said earlier, but the beauty of this is that when we eat the oil, our bodies convert it into a form that is deadly to troublesome microbes yet remains harmless to us.

All dietary oils, including coconut, are composed of triglycerides. Triglycerides are nothing more than three fatty acids hooked together to a glycerol molecule. When oil is eaten, the triglycerides break apart into diglycerides (two fatty acids joined by a glycerol), monoglycerides (one fatty acid attached to a glycerol), and free fatty acids. It is the monoglycerides and free fatty acids that have the antimicrobial properties. The most active are lauric acid and capric acid and their monoglycerides—monolaurin and monocaprin.

In regard to their antimicrobial properties, the monoglycerides and free fatty acids are active, and the diglycerides and triglycerides are inactive. The antimicrobial properties of coconut oil (which consists of triglycerides), therefore, become active only when ingested or otherwise converted into free fatty acids or monoglycerides.

Coconut and palm kernel oils are by far the richest natural sources of this supernutrient, which makes up about 50 percent of their fat content. Milk fat and butter are a distant second, having about 3 percent. These are the only food sources we have that contain significant amounts of lauric acid. Unlike the tropical oils, all vegetable oils are completely deficient in this and other MCFAs.

Lauric acid was first identified in the fruit and seed of the bay laurel tree, which grows in the Mediterranean region. The healing properties of this oil were recognized in ancient times. In Italy, France, Greece, Turkey, and Morocco the oil was used as a folk medicine to improve digestion, as a salve for bladder and skin diseases, and to provide protection against insect stings. It wasn't until the 1950s and 1960s that scientists began to unlock its healing secrets. Although laurel seeds contain 40 percent lauric acid, coconut and palm kernel oils provide a more abundant source. The medical research on lauric acid and other MCFAs is derived predominantly from the tropical oils.

Because of the many health benefits derived from lauric acid, researchers have recently been experimenting with ways to increase the amount of it available in our foods. They have been working with a variety of plants in an effort to increase their lauric acid content. Recently scientists have genetically engineered a new variety of canola called laurate canola that contains 36 percent lauric acid. In time this new canola may wind up being used in a variety of foods.

Lipid-Coated Microorganisms Killed by Lauric Acid	
LIPID-COATED VIRUSES	LIPID-COATED BACTERIA
HIV	Listeria monocytogenes
Measles virus	Helicobacter pylori
Herpes simplex virus	Hemophilus influenzae
Herpes viridae	Chlamydia pneumoniae
Sarcoma virus	Staphylococcus aureus
Syncytial virus	Streptococcus agalactiae
Human lymphotropic virus (Type 1)	Groups A, B, F, and G streptococci
Vesicular stomatitis virus (VSV)	Gram-positive organisms
Visna virus	Gram-negative organisms (if pretreated with chelator)
Cytomegalovirus	
Epstein-Barr virus	
Influenza virus	
Leukemia virus	
Pneumonovirus	
Hepatitis C virus	

The research demonstrating the many health benefits of the medium-chain fatty acids and their monoglycerides has been so compelling that companies are now marketing dietary supplements containing these products. Sold under many different brand names, Lauricidin® is a monolaurin supplement currently available from some health food stores and health care professionals. Dozens of health care clinics in the United States are actively using these supplements to treat patients and are achieving extraordinary success. For example, HIV-infected individuals using these supplements under clinical supervision have reported significant improvement in health. Most monolaurin supplements come in 300-milligram capsules.

Dietary supplements and genetically engineered vegetable oils are two ways in which the food and health industry is trying to increase our exposure to lauric acid. By far the best and richest natural sources of lauric acid are coconuts and coconut oil. For instance, 1 tablespoon of dried shredded coconut contains about 2 grams of lauric acid. A tablespoon of pure coconut oil contains 7 grams. Besides lauric acid, coconut products also contain other MCFAs, such as capric acid (7 percent) and caprylic acid (8 percent), both of which also have many beneficial effects on health that may be lacking in noncoconut sources.

This is an exciting area of research because it involves a readily available food source that can be used to both treat and prevent infectious illness. Wouldn't it be more pleasant to eat your favorite foods cooked in coconut oil to fight an infection rather than choke down a handful of antibiotics and suffer with their side effects? Eating a pizza made with coconut oil or a pudding made of coconut milk sounds a lot more appetizing than swallowing a bunch of nasty-tasting pills. Such a scenario may be possible. Researchers are currently working on formulations derived from the MCFAs in coconut oil to produce concentrated antimicrobial dietary supplements and pharmaceuticals.

HEALING APPLICATIONS

The potential uses of coconut oil for treating and preventing a wide assortment of infections is truly astounding, ranging from the flu to life-threatening conditions such as AIDS. Treating individuals infected with HIV, the virus that causes AIDS, by feeding them MCFAs has recently shown great promise, and research is now underway in this area. Eating coconut oil may be a simple solution to many illnesses we face today. Laboratory tests have shown that the MCFAs found in coconut oil are effective in destroying viruses that cause influenza, measles, herpes, mononucleosis, hepatitis C, and AIDS; bacteria that can cause stomach ulcers, throat infections, pneumonia, sinusitis, earache, rheumatic fever, dental cavities, food poisoning, urinary tract infections, meningitis, gonorrhea, and toxic shock syndrome; fungi and yeast that lead to ringworm, candida, and thrush; and parasites that can cause intestinal infections such as giardiasis.

The marvelous thing about using coconut oil to treat or prevent these conditions is that while it is deadly to disease-causing microorganisms, it is harmless to humans. The fatty acids that make coconut oil so effective against germs are the same ones nature has put into mother's milk to protect children. Human breast milk and the milk of other mammals all contain small amounts of MCFAs. This is why butter, which is concentrated milk fat, also contains MCFA. Milk with its medium-chain fatty acids protects the newborn baby from harmful germs at its most vulnerable time in life while its immune system is still developing. This is one of the reasons why coconut oil or MCFAs are added to infant formula. A mother who consumes coconut oil will have more MCFAs in her milk to help protect and nourish her baby. If it's safe enough for a newborn baby, it is safe enough for us. Nature made MCFAs to nourish and protect us against infectious illnesses.

Medical researchers develop marvelous synthetic drugs to fight infections, but all of them are accompanied by undesirable side effects.

Some are highly toxic. Coconut oil is nature's own antimicrobial weapon and, as a food that has withstood the test of time, is totally safe. While drugs may be necessary to treat certain illnesses, if you regularly eat coconut oil your chances of being infected with those illnesses should be greatly reduced.

Unlike most flu viruses, the virus that causes the common cold (rhinovirus) does not have a lipid coat and therefore is not vulnerable to the action of MCFAs. Cold and flu symptoms are often very similar, and it is difficult to tell which infection is present. In either case, however, coconut oil may be beneficial. Infections of any type depress the immune system, often allowing other germs to multiply, compounding the problem. If the infection is caused by a cold, the MCFAs will help kill these other troublesome microorganisms, thus relieving stress on the immune system and allowing it to more effectively fight the cold virus.

As research continues, coconut oil may prove to be one of the best internal antimicrobial substances available without a doctor's prescription. Simply adding coconut oil to your daily diet may provide you with substantial protection from a wide range of infectious illnesses. If you feel you are coming down with the flu, eating dried coconut or foods prepared with coconut oil may help you fight off the infection. If you have children, it may be the way to protect them against many childhood illness such as earaches and measles. Along with good dental hygiene, it might help to protect young teeth from developing cavities and periodontal disease. Eating something as ordinary as a pizza made with coconut oil may be one of the healthiest things you can do for yourself and your children.

BACTERIA

Until the discovery of antibiotics, medical science had little at its disposal to fight bacterial infections; all doctors could really do was make the patient as comfortable as possible while the body battled the disease.

Table 3.1. Bacteria Killed by Medium-Chain Fatty Acids

BACTERIUM	DISEASES CAUSED
Streptococcus	Throat infections, pneumonia, sinusitis, earache, rheumatic fever, dental cavities
Staphylococcus	Staph infection, food poisoning, urinary tract infections, toxic shock syndrome
Neisseria	Meningitis, gonorrhea, pelvic inflammatory disease
Chlamydia	Genital infections, lymphogranuloma venereum, conjunctivitis, parrot fever pneumonia, periodontitis
Helicobacter pyloris	Stomach ulcers
Gram-positive organisms	Anthrax, gastroenteritis, botulism, tetanus

Drugs have now become the standard weapon against disease-causing bacteria, but there are some natural products—foods and herbs—that also exhibit antibiotic properties and that have been used for generations with some degree of success. One of these is coconut oil.

The fatty acids found in coconut are powerful antibiotics. They are known to kill bacteria that can cause numerous illnesses. Table 3.1 lists some of the bacteria that MCFAs are effective against and the common diseases these organisms cause.

The standard treatment for all these bacterial infections is to use antibiotics, and this may be necessary in life-threatening situations. It is conceivable that instead of taking a drug for every single infection, we could simply eat foods that will kill these organisms. Onions, garlic, and echinacea are edible plants that are commonly used for this purpose already. Coconut appears to be another food that can serve this purpose, perhaps far better than any of the other natural antibiotics.

Take a look at stomach ulcers, for example. A recent analysis estimated that 90 percent of all stomach ulcers are caused by the *H. pyloris* bacterium and not excess acid, as was once believed. And MCFAs kill *H. pyloris.* In order to treat stomach ulcers there may come a time when your doctor will simply recommend eating more foods cooked in coconut oil. Using the oil regularly may even prevent the infection altogether. This may also be true for ear infections, pneumonia, food poisoning, and a host of other infectious illnesses. This is an exciting possibility that needs to be investigated more thoroughly. You don't need to wait 5 or 10 years, however, for the research to be completed before you can benefit from using coconut oil; because it's safe to use, you can add it to your diet now without fear.

One of the drawbacks to using antibiotics is that they generally kill a variety of bacteria both good and bad. Our intestines are the home to many "friendly" bacteria that cause no harm and are, in fact, necessary for good health. These friendly bacteria help digest nutrients, synthesize important vitamins (such as vitamin K) that are essential for our well-being, and compete for space with pathogenic or disease-causing bacteria and yeasts. A healthy human will have abundant intestinal bacteria, which prevent disease-causing troublemakers such as candida. Candida is a single-celled fungus or yeast cell that typically inhabits the intestinal tract. As long as good bacteria outnumber the candida and keep it under control, this yeast poses little threat.

When people take antibiotics, these good bacteria are often killed along with the disease-causing ones. This leaves yeast, such as candida, which is not affected by antibiotics, to grow unrestrained, proliferating and overrunning the intestinal tract. The consequence is a yeast overgrowth or infection. Such infections can last for years, causing a wide variety of symptoms ranging from headaches to digestive problems. Often people have systemic candida infections without even knowing it. This is why antifungal medications or probiotics should be taken whenever antibiotics are used. A probiotic supports the growth of friendly bacteria but not the disease-causing kind.

• YEAST AND FUNGI

Norma Galante, a Boston college student, went to her local medical clinic complaining of vaginal itching and a slight discharge. The physician took a culture of the discharge and examined it under the microscope. He diagnosed a mild bacterial infection and prescribed an antibiotic.

When Norma took the medication, however, it only made the symptoms worse. She went back to the doctor, and he gave her another antibiotic. It didn't work either. She tried again, and again, but he couldn't find a medication that would help. "I kept going back to the clinic, and the doctors kept prescribing different antibiotics," Norma says. Out of frustration, the physicians finally prescribed a topical anticandida cream to see if that would be of any help. While candida is not affected by antibiotics, it can be treated topically with antifungal creams and suppositories. Her symptoms subsided. She felt relieved. At last, she thought, her problem was solved.

Yeast infections are persistent and often recur, as was the case with Norma. It wasn't long before she had another infection. The medications she used seemed to relieve the symptoms, but within a few months they would flare up again. Before long she began to develop other fungal infections like athlete's foot and skin rashes (ringworm). Fungal infections of one sort or another became an ongoing nuisance. She felt chronically fatigued. Everything she did seemed to tire her. She became depressed. "The doctors didn't have any answers," she recalls. "To them I had a minor problem, but I was living with the itching and the fatigue every day; it wasn't a minor problem for me."

After receiving little help from her doctors, she began searching for an answer herself. She scoured health food stores for books and information on yeast infections. After studying these materials she realized she was suffering from a systemic or entire body candida infection. She cut sugar out of her diet and began taking a dietary supplement derived from coconut oil called caprylic acid. It worked! Both the vaginal yeast and skin infections healed. Without the constant strain of fighting the infection, her energy returned. She was able to function normally again without feeling constantly fatigued. "I was so relieved to find something that brought my energy back," she says.

One of the most widespread health problems in Western society is caused by the fungus *Candida albacans*. Many women are familiar with this troublesome pest because it is a common cause of vaginal yeast infections. It is also the same organism that causes oral thrush and diaper rash in babies. Candida is a single-celled fungus or yeast cell that inhabits the intestinal tract and mucous membranes of every living person on the earth. Within days after birth, newborns are infected and have a budding colony living in their digestive tract. Normally, competition from friendly bacteria and the cleansing action of our immune system keeps candida numbers low and prevents them from causing any adverse health problems. But when the immune system is compromised or when friendly bacteria in our gut are killed by taking antibiotics, a candida infection can quickly flare up. A single course of antibiotics can lead to a raging candida infection. Approximately 75 percent of women experience vaginal yeast infections at one time or another.

Vaginal yeast infections are typically treated as if they were only localized in one area of the body. Many people, however, have systemic infections in which candida grows out of control overrunning the digestive tract and affecting the entire body, including the reproductive system. Systemic yeast infections, called candidiasis (or yeast syndrome), affect the entire body and can afflict men as well as women. Symptoms are numerous and varied (see table 3.2), and even doctors have difficulty identifying the problem.

Because it is not easy to identify, hundreds of thousands of women and men are plagued with candidiasis without even realizing it. Vaginal yeast infections or oral yeast infections (thrush) can be identified by the white discharge they produce. Recurring vaginal yeast infections are one of the signs of a systemic infection. But you can have candidiasis without an active vaginal yeast infection. Anyone who has taken antibiotics, birth control pills, steroids, or immunosuppressive drugs is at high risk of having a

Table 3.2. Problems Commonly Associated
with Systemic Candida Infections

General	Fatigue, headache, digestive problems, joint pains, depression, memory loss, irritability, allergies
Women	Persistent vaginitis, menstrual irregularities, recurrent bladder problems
Men	Persistent or recurrent jock itch or athlete's foot, prostatitis, impotence
Children	Ear infections, hyperactivity, behavior and learning problems

Source: W. Crook, *The Yeast Connection* (1986)

systemic yeast infection, even if no noticeable symptoms are evident. Typical symptoms also include fatigue, depression, allergy symptoms, and recurring fungal skin infections (athlete's foot, jock itch, ringworm, etc.).

Skin fungus can afflict any part of the body from the head to the toe. Dry, flaky skin that persists despite the use of hand lotion and skin creams could very well be a fungal infection. Often what people call psoriasis is really a fungal infection. Dandruff is caused, in part, by skin fungus. Preadolescent children are the primary victims of scalp ringworm (tinea capitis), a skin fungus similar to athlete's foot. Not until puberty do glands secrete oil-containing MCFAs that help protect the scalp from skin fungus (see chapter 6 for more information on skin health).

HEALING FUNGAL AND YEAST INFECTIONS WITH COCONUT OIL

One of the most potent nondrug or natural yeast-fighting substances is caprylic acid, a medium-chain fatty acid derived from coconut oil. Caprylic acid in capsule form is commonly sold as a dietary supplement in health food stores. It is very effective against candida and other forms of fungi. It is even effective mixed with a little coconut oil or vitamin E oil as a topical application for fungal skin infections. I've seen fungal infections that have lasted for months clear up in a matter of days using caprylic acid and a little coconut oil. It works just as effectively inside the body, killing fungi without the least bit of harm.

Polynesian women who eat their traditional coconut-based diet rarely, if ever, get yeast infections. Only in more temperate climates where processed vegetable oils are the main source of dietary fat are yeast infections, skin fungus, acne, and other skin infections big problems. Lauric acid, found in coconut oil, kills lipid-coated bacteria but does not appear to harm the friendly intestinal bacteria. The MCFAs also have antifungal properties, so not only will they kill disease-causing bacteria and leave good bacteria alone but also they will kill candida and other fungi in the intestinal tract, further supporting a healthy intestinal environment. Eating coconut oil on a regular basis, as the Polynesians do, helps to keep candida and other harmful microorganisms at bay.

The efficiency of caprylic acid is reportedly so favorable that many supplement manufacturers put it in their products used to fight systemic and vaginal yeast infections. John P. Trowbridge, M.D., president of the American College for the Advancement of Medicine and author of *The Yeast Syndrome,* highly recommends caprylic acid as an aid to fight systemic candida infections.

The only effective cure for candidiasis has been dietary changes and medications. Caprylic acid is a natural yeast fighter that has been used very successfully in place of the drugs. Caprylic acid is often sold in combination with antifungal herbs in dietary supplements designed to help those with yeast infections. Caprinex (Nature's Way), Capricin (Professional Specialties), Mycostat (P & D Nutrition), and Caprystatin (Ecological Formulas) are the names of some of the anticandida supplements available.

PARASITES

There are two general groups of parasites. One consists of worms such as tapeworms and roundworms. The second category is the protozoa: one-celled organisms. Parasites infect the intestines of both humans and animals and can cause a great deal of intestinal distress. We often associate parasites with Third World countries and poor sanitation, but parasites are a problem everywhere, even in North America. In countries where sanitation is a priority, people mistakenly assume that no problem exists and they don't need to worry. But parasites are everywhere, waiting for the opportunity to latch onto an unsuspecting host. Backpackers have long been aware of the danger of drinking water from streams and lakes. Open water, even in the backcounty, is often contaminated with parasites waiting for a host.

Tap water can also be a source of contamination. The water treatment process doesn't remove all contaminants and parasites. Single-celled organisms such as cryptosporidium and giardia are particularly troublesome because they often slip through water purification treatment unharmed; since these organisms are protected by a tough outer coat, the chlorine added to municipal water supplies to kill germs has little effect on them. Because of their small size, very fine filters are needed to trap them, and complete elimination of these parasites from tap water isn't possible. Drinking-water regulations are designed to reduce but not necessarily eliminate parasite contamination; so even water systems that meet government standards may not be free of parasites. Water supplies must be constantly monitored to detect levels above acceptable limits, but even then the potential exists for giardia infection. The most susceptible are those who have a weak immune system that is incapable of mounting an effective defense against the organism. This is seen mostly in the very young and the elderly and those afflicted with immune-suppressing illnesses such as AIDS.

Two parasites, giardia and cryptosporidium, normally live in the digestive tracts of many mammals. Public water supplies can become infected with these organisms when they are contaminated by sewage or animal waste. Cryptosporidium is believed to be in 65 to 97 percent of the nation's surface waters (rivers, lakes, and streams), according to the CDC. About half of our tap water comes from treated surface water. Giardia is a much bigger problem. It ranks among the top 20 infectious diseases that cause the greatest morbidity in Africa, Asia, and Latin America, and it is also the most common parasite diagnosed in North America. The CDC estimates that two million Americans contract giardiasis every year.

Although you may not hear about it, outbreaks occur all the time, usually in smaller cities and occasionally in large metropolitan areas. Unsafe water is an embarrassment to the water department of any city, and sometimes officials are unwilling to admit that a problem exists until it's too late. Giardia is commonly found in the pretreated water system used by some 40 million Americans and has caused epidemics in several small cities. This was apparently what happened in Milwaukee, Wisconsin, in 1993. A breakdown in water sanitation permitted cryptosporidium to contaminate the city's drinking water for a week. As a result, 100 people died and 400,000 suffered with the stomach cramps, diarrhea, and fever that are characteristic of the parasite. Recent outbreaks have occurred in cities in California, Colorado, Montana, New York, Pennsylvania, and Massachusetts, to name just a few.

Giardia can live in a variety of water sources: streams, ponds, puddles, tap water, and swimming pools. Infection is spread by contact with an infected source. You don't have to drink contaminated water to become infected. Giardiasis can spread by sexual contact, poor personal hygiene, hand-to-mouth contact, and food handlers who don't wash their hands thoroughly. If your hands are exposed to contaminated water, animals, people, or feces (e.g., litter boxes, diapers), the infection could spread to you. Shoes can come in contact with animal droppings and bring it inside the home. Veterinary studies have shown that up to 13 percent of dogs are infected. Any pet can become a source of infection for humans, although it may not show signs of infection.

A study at Johns Hopkins Medical School a few years ago showed antibodies against giardia in 20 percent of randomly chosen blood samples from patients in the hospital. This means that at least 20 percent of these patients had been infected with giardia at some time in their lives and had mounted an immune response against the parasite. Giardia is rampant in day-care centers. A study in 1983 showed that 46 percent of those who were infected were associated with day-care centers or had contact with diaper-age children. It is estimated that 20 to 30 percent of workers in day-care centers harbor giardia. In a study done in Denver, Colorado, with 236 children attending day-care centers, 38 (16 percent) were found to be infected.

Symptoms of infection vary. It is often misdiagnosed and mistreated because its symptoms are similar to those of a number of other conditions, including the flu, irritable bowel syndrome, allergies, and chronic fatigue syndrome. In acute cases, symptoms are usually most severe and can include any of the following (listed in order of prevalence).

- Diarrhea
- Malaise (a sense of ill-being)
- Weakness
- Abdominal cramps
- Weight loss
- Greasy, foul-smelling stools
- Nausea
- Headaches
- Anorexia
- Abdominal bloating
- Flatulence
- Constipation
- Vomiting
- Fever

Infection can persist for weeks or months if left untreated. Some people undergo a more chronic phase that can last for many months. Chronic cases are characterized by loose stools and increased abdominal gassiness with cramping, depression, fatigue, and weight loss. Some people may have some symptoms and not others, while some may not have any symptoms at all.

Even if giardia is diagnosed and treated, it can damage the intestinal lining, causing chronic health problems that persist for years after the parasite is gone. Food allergies, including lactose (milk) intolerance, can develop. Damaged intestinal tissues become leaky. This is often referred to as leaky gut syndrome. Toxins, bacteria, and incompletely digested foods are able to pass through the intestinal wall into the bloodstream, initiating an immune response. Sinus congestion, aches and pains, headaches, swelling, and inflammation—all typical symptoms of allergies—are the result.

Loss of intestinal integrity can lead to the gastrointestinal discomfort known as irritable bowel syndrome (IBS). Dr. Leo Galland, an expert in gastrointestinal disease, demonstrated that out of a group of 200 patients with chronic diarrhea, constipation, abdominal pain, and bloating, half were infected with giardia. Most of these patients had been told they had irritable bowel syndrome. He notes that parasitic infection is a common event among patients with chronic gastrointestinal symptoms, and many people are given a diagnosis of irritable bowel syndrome without a thorough evaluation.

Another consequence of poor intestinal integrity is fatigue resulting from malabsorption of important nutrients. If the condition persists, it can lead to chronic fatigue syndrome. A giardia infection can be so draining on the immune system that it causes fatigue. Again the cause is often misdiagnosed. A giardia epidemic in Placerville, California, for example, was mysteriously followed by an epidemic of chronic fatigue syndrome. In 1991 Dr. Galland and his colleagues published a study of 96 patients with chronic fatigue and demonstrated active giardia infection in 46 percent. In another study of 218 patients whose chief complaint was chronic fatigue, Dr. Galland found that 61 patients were infected with giardia. His conclusion is that giardia may be an important cause of chronic fatigue syndrome.

COCONUT OIL DEFENDS AGAINST PARASITES

Coconut oil may provide an effective defense against many troublesome parasites, including giardia. Research has shown that, like bacteria and fungi, giardia and possibly other protozoa can't stand up against MCFAs. By using coconut oil and other coconut products every day, you may be able to destroy giardia before it can establish a foothold. In doing so you also eliminate the possibility of developing food allergies, chronic fatigue, and other related symptoms. If you're currently troubled with these conditions, coconut oil used liberally with meals may provide a source of relief. Because MCFAs are quickly absorbed by the tissues and converted into energy, it seems logical that those suffering from chronic fatigue would gain a great deal of benefit. Foods prepared with coconut oil, or even fresh coconut, make a great energy booster without adversely affecting blood sugar.

Another possible use for coconut is for the removal of intestinal worms. In India, in fact, it has been used to get rid of tapeworms and is rubbed into the scalp as a treatment to remove head lice. In one study it was reported that treatment with dried coconut, followed by magnesium sulfate (a laxative), caused 90 percent parasite expulsion after 12 hours. The authors of some pet books apparently have had success with coconut and recommend feeding animals ground coconut as a means of expelling intestinal parasites. Tapeworms, lice, giardia, candida, bacteria, viruses, and germs of all sorts can be eliminated, or at least held in check, with coconut oil; it is one of the best natural remedies you can use.

A SHIELD AGAINST DISEASE

Tropical diseases such a malaria and yellow fever have plagued human-kind for centuries. Throughout history, whenever people from moderate climates have settled or traveled in areas covered by tropical jungles, they've been plagued by disease. Even today people who travel in these areas must be cautious.

The curious thing about this is that the people who are living in these areas don't succumb to disease. Researchers have been unable to find any genetic reason for their resistance. Locals who move out of the area and return several years later are often susceptible to disease just like any other outsider.

I believe the local people are protected because of the type of food they eat, in particular coconuts. It is in these tropical climates that coconuts grow abundantly and serve as a valuable food source for the local inhabitants. It is as if the coconut were put there on purpose not only to serve as a source of food but to protect people from disease. In his studies of African natives, Dr. Weston A. Price noted in his book *Nutrition and Physical Degeneration* that those who consumed traditional local foods did not suffer from insect-borne diseases such as malaria. Tropical climates are breeding grounds for all types of disease-causing organisms, yet indigenous peoples have lived in these places generation after generation without problem. Only those people from other climates, who eat virtually no coconut or other native plants, have a difficult time.

Herbalists have noted for years that in regions where certain diseases are common, medicinal plants grow that can cure these diseases. This is why every culture in the world has a form of traditional medicine based on the use of local herbs. The people who live in the tropics where coconut grows are protected to some extent from malaria, yellow fever, and other common infectious organisms. The people in Panama have discovered the importance of coconut as a means of staying healthy.

When they feel an illness coming on they increase their consumption of coconut, particularly the milk and the oil. Likewise, Africans in tropical areas will drink palm kernel oil whenever they get sick.

Before the onset of World War II, American contractors went to the Panama Canal to build airstrips, submarine bases, and barracks for the military. Workers from the city, as well as natives from the jungles of Central America and the Caribbean, came in to provide the labor. Coconut was an important source of food for these natives. In 1940 many of them still lived a relatively isolated existence. Many spoke neither Spanish nor English. Local labor was preferred, because over the years it was noticed that indigenous people were more resistant to disease and worked harder. One of the contractors, William Bockus, Jr., observed: "There were two striking differences between these Indians and the majority of the other workers. They were never sick and they were slim and trim. These guys would work steadily all day long in the swamps in mud and rain without complaint. Foremen had to tell them to take rest periods, believe it or not. They also never missed a day's work." This is a far cry from the situation just a few years earlier, when malaria and yellow fever devastated the French and American workers who built the Panama Canal.

In my opinion, the coconut is one of God's greatest health foods and, when consumed as part of your regular diet, can protect you against a host of infectious illnesses. Eating coconuts and coconut oil can provide you with some degree of protection from a wide variety of disease-causing organisms. Coconut oil may not be able to cure all disease, but it can help prevent many illnesses, relieve stress on the immune system, and allow the body to resist disease better. A person who is aware of the health benefits of coconut oil but doesn't use it is like the person who doesn't wear a seat belt when driving. You've got a seat belt that can protect you from a number of nasty diseases. It would be foolish not to take advantage of it.

5

EAT FAT, LOSE WEIGHT

The world's population is growing—at the waist. More people are overweight now than ever before. The number of overweight people has greatly increased over the past few decades, and particularly over the last 10 years. According to the CDC, the number of obese people in the United States has exploded over the past decade from 12 percent of the total population to 17.9 percent. In the United States, 55 percent of the population is overweight; one in four adults is considered obese. As much as 25 percent of all teenagers are overweight. Even our kids are becoming fatter. The number of overweight children has more than doubled in the past 30 years. Figures (and waistlines) are similar in the United Kingdom, Germany, and many other affluent countries.

A person is considered obese if his or her weight is 20 percent or more above the maximum desirable weight. Over the past decade obesity has increased by 70 percent among people aged 18–29. For those 30–39 years old, it has increased 50 percent. All other age groups have likewise experienced a dramatic increase in weight.

Medical problems can escalate the battle of the bulge into a full-scale war. Being overweight increases risk for gallbladder disease, osteoarthritis, diabetes, heart disease, and early death. If you are overweight, losing some pounds could be one of the healthiest things you can do for yourself.

If you are like most people, you've noticed a gradual increase in your waistline over the years. Most of us do. I'm no exception. I never considered myself exactly fat, just a little pudgy here and there. For several years I tried to lose some of this excess weight, and I believed that I could. For years I kept several pair of my favorite pants that were too small for me. I knew I would lose enough weight to fit back into them.

Well, I tried. I reduced my fat intake, ate less food, and was hungry all the time. I thought I ate healthfully. My meals were well balanced with the different food groups. I avoided saturated fat and used the so-called healthy oils like margarine and liquid vegetable oil for all food preparation needs. The only thing dieting accomplished was to make me miserable. My stomach rumbled and complained constantly. I felt denied. It was depressing. Finally, I just gave up; it wasn't worth the trouble. I gave up on weight-reducing diets. I came to the conclusion that I would never lose any weight permanently. I gathered up all the clothes that wouldn't fit me and tossed them out.

But as I learned more about diet, health, and coconut oil, I realized I was eating the wrong kinds of oil. Instead of going on another diet, I replaced the processed vegetable oils I was eating with coconut oil. I used butter instead of margarine. I ate fewer sweets and more fiber. I didn't reduce the amount of food I was eating, and I probably ate more calories than I had before because I began eating more fat, in the form of coconut oil.

A strange thing happened. I didn't expect it to happen, and I didn't even notice it until months later. My pants were becoming looser. I was able to cinch my belt up tighter. I hadn't weighed myself for some time, but when I stepped back on the scale, I found that I had lost about 20 pounds. I was shocked because I wasn't dieting. I wasn't trying to lose weight, I was just trying to eat healthier. The weight had just came off on its own. I regretted that I'd tossed out all my favorite pants.

I have been eating this way now for several years. I don't feel deprived. I eat foods cooked in fat. I eat desserts containing fat. But the fat I eat is almost exclusively coconut oil. The 20 pounds are still gone. I am at my ideal weight for my height and bone structure. I found a way of

Health Problems Associated with Obesity

Abdominal hernias

Gout

Hypertension

Varicose veins

Diabetes

Cancer

Arthritis

Coronary heart disease

Respiratory problems

Atherosclerosis

Gastrointestinal disorders

Gynecological irregularities

eating that wasn't like a weight-loss diet because it worked without my trying. It was great. I look better and feel better about myself.

This chapter is for all who want to lose unwanted weight permanently without struggling with weight-reducing diets. You don't need to diet to lose weight; instead you need to make wise food choices. Your food can be just as tasty and satisfying yet still be healthy and weight-reducing.

WHY WE COUNT CALORIES

What makes people fat? Basically it's consuming more food than our bodies need. The food we eat is converted into energy—measured in calories—which powers metabolic functions and physical activity. Any excess calories are converted into fat and packed away into fat cells to produce the cellulite on our legs, the spare tire around our middle, and the oversized seat cushions on our backsides. So the more we eat, the bigger we get.

The rate at which the body uses calories for these maintenance activities is called the basal metabolic rate (BMR). It is equivalent to the number of calories a person would expend while lying down, inactive but awake. Any physical activity, no matter how simple, would require additional calories. At least two-thirds of the calories we use every day go to fuel basic metabolic functions.

Each of us has a different BMR. Many factors determine your BMR and the amount of calories your body needs and uses. Young people require more calories than older people. Physically active people use more than less active ones. People who are fasting, starving, or even dieting use *fewer* calories. Overweight people use fewer calories than lean or muscular people. These last two situations are unwelcome news to people who are overweight and dieting. It means they have to eat even less to see a change.

The two most influential factors over which we have control in determining body weight are calorie consumption and physical activity. Let's look at an example of how food consumption and exercise affect weight. A 150-pound man with a sedentary job, such as a computer keyboard operator, needs about 1,600 calories for basic metabolic functions and another 800 calories for daily physical activities. He would need to consume a total of 2,400 (1,600 plus 800) calories a day to maintain his body weight. Weight gain could be caused by two factors: (1) if he eats more than 2,400 calories, all the additional calories will be converted into fat, and he gains weight; and (2) if he becomes less active than he already is, his body will use fewer calories and turn the excess into fat. But our man could also lose weight two ways: (1) if he doesn't get 2,400 calories from his diet, his body will produce them from the breakdown of fatty tissues; and (2) if he exercises, his body will draw on his fat stores to provide the energy for his increased activity level.

A healthy calorie intake will vary from person to person, depending on activity level, and from men to women. A man with a job that requires moderate activity, such as janitorial work, needs about 2,600–2,800 calories a day to maintain his weight. For a heavy job, such as bricklaying, one needs about 2,800–3,200 calories a day. An average-sized male needs between 2,200 and 3,200 calories a day, depending on his level of physical activity. Women are generally smaller and have less muscle mass than men, so they need fewer calories—about 2,000–2,800.

LOSE WEIGHT QUICK?

You've seen the advertisements. "I lost fifty pound in four weeks." "I went from a size eighteen to a size eight in thirty days!" All sorts of diets claim that you can lose weight "quickly." Is it really possible to lose weight this fast? Let's take a look at the facts.

A pound of body fat stores about 3,500 calories. To lose it, you must reduce your calorie intake by 3,500. On average, a reduction of 500 calories a day (3,500/week) brings about a weight loss of one pound a week. A reduction of 1,000 calories a day equates to a loss of 2 pounds a week. To eliminate 1,000 calories a day, an average-sized person would need to reduce his or her food intake by nearly half. That's a big reduction! What this means is that true fat loss takes time. You cannot lose 50 pounds of fat in six weeks! It's just not possible unless you are very obese and don't consume anything except water. Six to 12 pounds is more realistic in this time frame.

Many people would disagree with this statement and claim that they lost 10 pounds in two weeks or some other short amount of time. But weight loss can be deceiving. A pound lost does not necessarily indicate a reduction in body fat. Quick changes in weight are not changes in fat but are due primarily to a loss of water. Look at the numbers. On average, we need about 2,500 calories a day to maintain current weight, whether we are over- or underweight. This is the amount needed just to stay even. Out of this number, two-thirds, or 1,667 calories, are needed just to power basic metabolic processes. A reduction of 1,000 calories a day is dramatic and borders on starvation because you would not even get enough calories to fuel these functions, let alone your daily activities.

This great a reduction in calories would also require you to drastically reduce the amount you eat each day, even if you chose low-calorie foods. At this drastic rate you would only lose 2 pounds of fat a week. In addition, you would be constantly hungry and fatigued due to a lack of energy. Claims in advertisements that somebody on a particular diet lost 10 pounds in one week or 40 pounds in four weeks or some other incredible figure may be true, but it wasn't fat they lost, it was muscle mass and water. In time, the water will be added back and weight will increase. If water isn't eventually replaced, it can lead to some very serious health problems caused by chronic dehydration.

In order to lose fat and excess weight permanently and healthfully, you need to do it slowly. The best way to lose weight is to make small adjustments in the types of foods you eat, increase your activity level, and stop worrying about counting calories or denying yourself. It can be done. And as I will soon show, adding coconut oil to your diet will make weight loss easier.

A BIG FAT PROBLEM

While some foods provide more calories than others, overeating any food will add additional pounds to one's waistline. There are three nutrients that give us energy, or calories—fat, protein, and carbohydrate. Every gram of protein we eat, whether it comes from meat or wheat, supplies our bodies with 4 calories. Carbohydrate, which is the primary energy source in vegetables, fruits, and grains, also supplies 4 calories per gram. Fat, however, supplies more than twice that—9 calories per gram. So you would need to eat more than twice as much protein or carbohydrate to get the same amount of calories you do from fat.

Reducing the amount of fat we eat is a logical way to reduce total calorie consumption and lose unwanted weight. But few people can stick to a low-fat or no-fat diet for long. Fats make food taste better and are necessary in the preparation of many dishes and baked goods. Statistics show that nearly all those who go on low-fat diets to lose weight regain the weight after a couple of years, often putting on more weight than they had before. Eliminating fat from the diet takes a tremendous amount of willpower and to be truly successful requires a lifelong commitment. Most of us aren't willing to eliminate fat from our diet for the rest of our lives.

In addition, fats are actually important food components without which we would suffer from nutrient deficiencies. It is through the fats in our food that we get the fat-soluble vitamins (A, D, E, and K and beta-carotene). Researchers are showing that these nutrients protect us from a myriad of diseases, including cancer and heart disease. Fat is required in our foods in order to obtain and absorb these nutrients. A low-fat diet can lead to nutrient deficiencies and increase the risk of numerous degenerative diseases.

Some fats are considered essential because our bodies cannot make them from other nutrients. This is why the American Heart Association, the National Heart, Lung, and Blood Institute, and other organizations all recommend that we get 30 percent of our daily calories from fat. In comparison, these organizations also recommend that we get only 12 percent of our calories from protein and that the rest should come from carbohydrates.

NOT ALL FATS ARE ALIKE

We have a dilemma here. Fat is, to put it bluntly, fattening. The more fat we eat, the more calories we consume, and the harder it is to lose weight. But if we cut down on fats, we also cut out the essential fatty acids and the fat-soluble vitamins.

What if there was a fat that had fewer calories than other fats and actually promoted better health—would you be interested? Sound like a pipe dream? It's not. There actually is a fat that can do this. That fat is found in coconut oil.

Replacing the fats you now eat with coconut oil may be the wisest decision you can make to lose excess body fat. We often think that the less fat we eat, the better. However, you don't necessarily need to reduce your fat intake; you simply need to choose a fat that is better for you—one that doesn't contribute to weight gain. You can lose unwanted body fat by eating more saturated fat (in the form of coconut oil) and less polyunsaturated fat (processed vegetable oils).

All fats, whether they are saturated or unsaturated, from a cow or from corn, contain the same number of calories. The MCFAs in coconut oil, however, contain a little less. Because of the small size of the fatty acids that make up coconut oil, they actually yield fewer calories than other fats. For example, MCT oil, which is derived from coconut oil and consists of 75 percent caprylic acid (C:8) and 25 percent capric acid (C:10), has an effective energy value of only 6.8 calories per gram. This is much less than the 9 calories per gram supplied by other fats. Coconut oil has at least 2.56 percent fewer calories per gram of fat than long-chain fatty acids. This means that if you use coconut oil in place of other oils, your calorie intake is lower.

This small reduction in calories is only part of the picture. The type of calories coconut oil contributes is in effect closer to that of carbohydrate because coconut oil is digested and processed differently from other fats.

COCONUT OIL PRODUCES ENERGY, NOT FAT

When people go on diets to lose weight, the foods that are restricted most are those that contain the most fat. Why is fat singled out? We know it is high in calories, but there is another reason. Because of the way it is digested and utilized in our bodies, it contributes the most to body fat. The fat we eat is the fat we wear—literally.

When we eat fat, it is broken down into individual fatty acids and repackaged into small bundles of fat and protein called lipoproteins.

These lipoproteins are sent into the bloodstream, where the fatty acids are deposited directly into our fat cells. Other nutrients, such as carbohydrate and protein, are broken down and used immediately for energy or tissue building. Only when we eat too much is the excess carbohydrate and protein converted into fat. As long as we eat enough to satisfy energy needs, fat in our food ends up as fat in our cells. Only between meals, when physical activity outpaces energy reserves, is fat removed from storage and burned for fuel.

However, MCFAs are digested and utilized differently. They are not packaged into lipoproteins and do not circulate in the bloodstream like other fats but are sent directly to the liver, where they are immediately converted into energy—just like a carbohydrate. But unlike carbohydrates, MCFAs do not raise blood sugar, so coconut oil is safe for diabetics. Many people report that coconut oil helps them control sugar cravings and reduces hypoglycemic symptoms. So when you eat coconut oil, the body uses it immediately to make energy rather than store it as body fat. As a consequence, you can eat much more coconut oil than you can other oils before the excess is converted into fat. It has been well documented in numerous dietary studies, using both animals and humans, that replacing LCFAs with MCFAs results in a decrease in body weight gain and a reduction in fat deposition.

These studies have scientifically verified that replacing traditional sources of dietary fat, which are composed primarily of LCFAs, with MCFAs yields meals with a lower effective calorie content. So MCFAs can be a useful tool in controlling weight gain and fat deposition. The simplest and best way to replace LCFAs with MCFAs is to use coconut oil in the preparation of your food.

METABOLIC ROLLER COASTER

Don't you hate them—those people who are as skinny as rails and eat like horses? They're full of pep and vitality, gorge themselves on all types of fattening foods, and never gain an ounce. You, on the other hand, eat a celery stick and immediately gain 5 pounds. Why is that? The answer is metabolism. Your basal metabolic rate is slower than theirs. They burn up more calories with the same amount of physical activity as you. They can eat more than you but weigh less. Wouldn't it be nice to increase your metabolic rate?

The best way you can rev up your metabolism is to exercise. When you exercise regularly, metabolism picks up. During exercise metabolism increases, and it remains elevated even when you're not exercising. A physically fit body also burns more calories than one that is not, because lean body tissue burns more calories than fatty tissue. So a person in good physical shape uses more calories. This is why one person can eat like a gorilla and look as skinny as a bird, while someone else can eat like a bird and still pack on weight.

Metabolism is also affected by the amount of food we eat. If we suddenly start to eat less, as when we diet, it signals to our bodies that there must be less food available, and as a means of self-preservation our BMR decreases to conserve energy. The slower metabolism also means that our bodies produce less energy, and so we become fatigued more easily.

Because dieting tends to make us feel hungry and tired all the time as our BMR drops in order to match the lowered intake of calories, in order to see a significant reduction in weight you must eat even less, essentially starving yourself, consuming fewer calories than your body actually needs for daily activities. If you are overweight and reduce your eating to just enough to match the amount of calories you use each day, you won't lose a thing. You will maintain your current weight level. In order to reduce, you must nearly starve yourself—*or* you must significantly increase your physical activity. Exercise is beneficial because it keeps your BMR normal or increases it so that your body burns more calories. If you combine exercise with dieting, you get the most weight-reducing effect because you lower your calorie intake and increase both your daily use of calories and your BMR.

DIETING MAKES YOU FAT

Someone once said, "Over the past several years I've lost two hundred pounds. If I'd kept it all off I would weigh minus twenty pounds." Many people can identify with this statement. Dieting hasn't helped. In fact, dieting can actually make you fat! How does it do that? After depriving yourself for a period of time in order to lose weight, you begin to ease up on the diet. Most people experience sensations of intense hunger and begin to eat at least as much as they ate before the diet started, if not more. The diet may have resulted in a loss of 10 or 15 pounds in the first few weeks, most of which was water. After you end the diet, your food cravings prompt you to eat and overeat. But now the calories you eat pack a heftier punch. Why? Because your BMR has decreased. The 800-calorie meal will have the same effect as, say, a 1,000-calorie meal. The result? You regain all the weight you lost and then some. By the time your BMR catches up, you're already overweight again. This time you weigh more than you ever did. With a lower metabolic rate, you burn less and less, and it becomes harder and harder to lose. When you do start eating again, you're more likely to store fat rather than burn it because you're burning it at a lower level.

Now bigger than ever, you may build up the courage to try dieting again. You again limit your calorie/food consumption and experience good results at first as your body sheds water. You hit a plateau when you've lost all the water your body is willing to give up, and your metabolism begins to drop. You become discouraged and start eating again. You regain all the weight you had lost and then some. With each new diet you end up gaining more and more weight.

Only those people who can carefully watch what they eat, stick to it, and exercise regularly keep the weight off permanently. Crash diets don't work. Lifestyle changes do.

A METABOLIC MARVEL

Wouldn't it be nice to be able to take a pill that would shift your metabolic rate into a higher gear? In a sense, that is what happens every time we eat. Food affects our BMR, and when we eat, many of our body's cells increase their activities to facilitate digestion and assimilation. This stimulation of cellular activity, known as diet-induced thermogenesis, uses about 10 percent of the total food energy taken in. Perhaps you have noticed, particularly on cool days, that you feel warmer after eating a meal. Your body's engines are running at a slightly higher rate, so more heat is produced. Different types of foods produce different thermogenic effects. Protein-rich foods such as meat increase thermogenesis and have a stimulatory or energizing effect on the body. But this is only true if you don't overeat. Overeating puts tremendous strain on the digestive system, which can drain your energy and make you feel tired. This is why we often feel sleepy after a big meal.

Protein has a much greater thermogenic effect than carbohydrate. This is why when people suddenly cut down on meat consumption or become vegetarians they often complain of a lack of energy, and it is one of the reasons high-protein diets promote weight loss—the increase in metabolism burns off more calories.

One food that can rev up your metabolism even more than protein is coconut oil. The MCFAs shift the body's metabolism into a higher gear, so to speak, so that you burn more calories. Because MCFAs increase the metabolic rate, coconut oil is a dietary fat that can actually promote weight loss! A dietary fat that takes off weight rather than putting it on is a strange concept indeed, but that is exactly what happens, so long as calories in excess of the body's needs are not consumed. The MCFAs are easily absorbed and rapidly burned and used as energy for metabolism, thus increasing metabolic activity and even burning LCFAs. So not only are medium-chain fatty acids burned for energy production, but also they encourage the burning of long-chain fatty acids as well.

Dr. Julian Whitaker, a well-known authority on nutrition and health, makes this analogy between the long-chain triglycerides and medium-chain triglycerides: "LCTs are like heavy wet logs that you put on a small campfire. Keep adding the logs, and soon you have more logs than fire. MCTs are like rolled-up newspaper soaked in gasoline. They not only burn brightly, but will burn up the wet logs as well" (Murray, 1996).

Research supports Dr. Whitaker's view. In one study, the thermo-genic (fat-burning) effect of a high-calorie diet containing 40 percent fat as MCFAs was compared to one containing 40 percent fat as LCFAs. The thermogenic effect of the MCFAs was almost twice as high as that of the LCFAs: 120 calories versus 66 calories. The researchers concluded that the excess energy provided by fats in the form of MCFAs would not be efficiently stored as fat but rather would be burned. A followup study demonstrated that MCFAs given over a six-day period can in-crease diet-induced thermogenesis by 50 percent.

In another study, researchers compared single meals of 400 calories composed of MCFAs or LCFAs. The thermogenic effect of MCFAs over six hours was three times greater than that of LCFAs. Researchers concluded that substituting MCFAs for LCFAs would produce weight loss as long as the calorie level remained the same.

Researchers can evaluate changes in metabolism by measuring en-ergy expenditure (the amount of calories used by the body). As metab-olism increases, the amount of energy, or number of calories, burned increases. In one study, energy expenditure was measured in volunteers before eating a meal containing MCTs and then afterward. It was found that in normal-weight individuals, energy expenditure increased by 48 percent. That means their metabolism had increased to the point that they were burning 48 percent more calories than normal. In obese sub-jects energy expenditure increased by an incredible 65 percent! So the more body fat a person has, the greater effect the oil has on metabolism.

This thermogenic or calorie-burning effect doesn't last for just one or two hours after a meal. Studies show that after eating a single meal containing MCTs, metabolism remains elevated for at least 24 hours! So when you eat a meal that contains coconut oil, your metabolism will increase and remain elevated for at least 24 hours. During this entire time you will have a higher level of energy and you will be burning calories at an accelerated rate.

Researchers at McGill University in Canada have found that if you replace all the oils in your diet that are made of long-chain triglycerides, such as soybean oil, canola oil, safflower oil, and the like, with an oil that contains MCTs, such as coconut oil, you can lose up to 36 pounds of excess fat a year. This is without changing your diet and without reducing the number of calories you eat. All you simply have to do to is get an oil change.

Adding coconut to your diet can be a great way to help you lose excess body fat. But keep in mind that even though coconut oil can speed

---

"I didn't have many expectations when I started using coconut oil a year ago. I was overweight, and resigned to it; diets just didn't work with me. In fact, in spite of a basically healthy diet I was steadily gaining weight over the years and decades. I was also using what I considered the healthy fats—polyunsaturated oils.

"After reading Bruce Fife's books on coconut oil I switched oils completely. I diligently read labels to avoid hydrogenated vegetable oils—and was amazed at how pervasive they are. I used coconut oil for all my cooking, and even added it to my tea.

"I lost 20 pounds in a matter of weeks, and, what's more important, my weight has stayed at this level for the whole year. Even at times of more indulgence, such as holidays and Christmas, I did not gain. I take coconut oil with me wherever I go and can't live without my daily dose! I'm convinced that it was the polyunsaturated oils that made me gain weight, and coconut oil that helped me lose it.

"Also, my energy is up; formerly I was prone to inactivity but now I can go all day. Another side effect—my dandruff has disappeared completely."

—*Sharon Maas*

up your metabolism, if you overeat you will still gain weight. The best way to lose weight with coconut oil is to add it to a sensible diet.

ENERGY AND METABOLISM

Eating foods containing MCFAs is like putting high-octane fuel into your car. The car runs more smoothly and gets better gas mileage. Likewise, with MCFAs, your body performs better because it has more energy and greater endurance. Because MCFAs are funneled directly to the liver and converted into energy, the body gets a boost of energy. And because MCFAs are easily absorbed by the energy-producing organelles of the cells, metabolism increases. This burst of energy has a stimulating effect on the entire body.

The fact that MCFAs digest immediately to produce energy and stimulate metabolism has led athletes to use them as a means to enhance exercise performance. Studies indicate this may be true. In one study, for example, investigators tested the physical endurance of mice who were given MCFAs in their daily diet against those that weren't. The study extended over a six-week period. The mice were subjected to a swimming endurance test every other day. They were placed in a pool of water with a constant current. The total swimming time until exhaustion was measured. On the first day there was little difference between the groups of mice. As the study progressed, the mice that had been fed MCFAs quickly began to outperform the others and continued to improve throughout the testing period. Tests such as this demonstrate that MCFAs have the ability to enhance endurance and exercise performance, at least in mice. Another study using human subjects supports the animal studies. In this study, conditioned cyclists were used. The cyclists pedaled at 70 percent of maximum for two hours, then immediately embarked on a 40-kilometer time trial ride (lasting about an additional hour) while drinking one of three beverages: an MCFA solution, a sports drink, or a sports drink/MCFA combination. The cyclists who drank the sports drink/MCFA mixture performed the best during the time trial.

The authors of the study theorized that the MCFAs gave the cyclists an additional source of energy, thus sparing glycogen stores. Glycogen, the energy stored in muscle tissue, would have been used up during the three-hour ride. The more glycogen in the muscles, the greater an athlete's endurance. So any substance that can conserve glycogen while providing energy would be useful to endurance athletes. In a followup study to test the glycogen-sparing theory, participants cycled at 60 percent of their maximum for three hours while drinking one of three beverages, as was done in the earlier study. Following the exercise, muscle glycogen levels were measured and found to be the same for all three groups. The conclusion was that MCFAs did not spare glycogen stores yet did improve performance. The improvement in performance was not due to glycogen sparing and must be attributed to some other mechanism.

Because of these and similar studies, many of the powdered sports drinks and energy bars sold at health food stores contain MCTs to provide a quick source of energy. The MCFAs most often used in sports drinks and energy bars are in the form of MCT oil. This ingredient is usually listed as "MCT" on food, supplement, and infant formula labels. Athletes and other active people looking for nutritional, nondrug methods to enhance exercise performance have begun using them.

Although many studies have shown that MCFAs boost energy and endurance, other studies have shown little or no effect, at least when MCFA mixtures are taken in a single oral dose. Studies generally show that a single oral dose has little measurable effect. In studies where animals were fed MCFAs as a part of their daily diet, however, the results were more significant. From this evidence it appears that the best way to increase energy and endurance is to consume MCFAs on a daily basis and not a single time just before or during competition.

It's easy to see why athletes would be interested in gaining greater endurance and energy, but what about nonathletes? What about people who diet and feel low in energy because of food restriction? The MCFAs can do the same for them. If eaten regularly, MCFAs can provide a boost in energy and performance of daily activities. Would you like to increase your energy level throughout the day? If you get tired in the middle of the day or feel you lack energy, adding coconut oil to your daily diet may provide you with a much-needed boost to help carry you through.

The boost in energy you get from coconut oil is not like the kick you get from caffeine; it's more subtle than that but longer lasting. As mentioned earlier, metabolism is elevated and remains so for at least 24 hours. During this time you will enjoy a slightly higher level of energy and vitality.

Besides increasing your energy level, there are other very important benefits of boosting your metabolic rate: it helps protect you from illness and speeds healing. When metabolism is increased, cells function at a higher rate of efficiency. They heal injuries quicker; old and diseased cells are replaced faster; and young, new cells are generated at an increased rate to replace worn-out ones. Even the immune system functions better.

Several health problems such as obesity, heart disease, and osteoporosis are more prevalent in those people who have slow metabolism. Any health condition is made worse if the metabolic rate is slower than normal, because cells can't heal and repair themselves as quickly. Increasing metabolic rate, therefore, provides an increased degree of protection from both degenerative and infectious illnesses.

THE SKINNY ON COCONUT OIL

Coconut oil contains the most concentrated natural source of MCFAs available. Substituting coconut oil for other vegetable oils in your diet will help promote weight loss. The use of refined vegetable oil actually promotes weight gain, not just from its calorie content but because of its harmful effects on the thyroid—the gland that controls metabolism. Polyunsaturated vegetable oils depress thyroid activity, thus lowering metabolic rate—just the opposite of coconut oil. Eating polyunsaturated oils, like soybean oil, will contribute more to weight gain than other fats, even more than beef tallow and lard. According to Ray Peat, Ph.D., an endocrinologist who specializes in the study of hormones, unsaturated oils block thyroid hormone secretion, its movement in the circulation, and the response of tissues to the hormone. When thyroid hormones are deficient, metabolism becomes depressed. Polyunsaturated oils are, in essence, high-calorie fats that encourage weight gain more than any other fats. If you wanted to lose weight, you would be better off eating lard, because lard doesn't interfere with thyroid function.

Farmers are always looking for ways to fatten their livestock because bigger animals bring bigger profits. Fats and oils are used as an additive in animal feed to quickly pack on weight in preparing them for market. Saturated fat seems like a good choice to fatten up livestock, so pig farmers tried to feed coconut products to their animals for this purpose, but when it was added to the animal feed, the pigs lost weight! Farmers found that the high polyunsaturated oil content of corn and soybeans quickly did what the coconut oil couldn't. Animals fed corn and soybeans packed on pounds quickly and easily. The reason these oils worked so well is that their oils suppressed thyroid function, decreasing the animals' metabolic rate. (Soybeans are particularly bad because of the goitrogens [antithyroid chemicals] they contain.) They could eat less food and gain more weight! Many people are in a similar situation. Every time we eat polyunsaturated oils, our thyroid gland is assaulted and loses its ability to function normally. Weight gain is one of the consequences.

6

BEAUTIFUL SKIN AND HAIR

For thousands of years, coconut oil has been used to make the skin soft and smooth and give hair a rich, shiny luster. Polynesian women are famed for their beautiful skin and hair, even though they are exposed to the hot blistering sun and chafing of the ocean breeze every day. As a skin lotion and hair conditioner, no other oil can compare.

Because coconut oil has a natural creamy texture, comes from a vegetable source, and is almost always free from pesticides and other chemicals and contaminants, it has been used for years in soaps, shampoos, creams, and other body-care products. Its small molecular structure allows for easy absorption, giving both the skin and hair a soft, smooth texture. It makes an ideal ointment for the relief of dry, rough, and wrinkled skin. Many people use it as a lip balm because it is safe and natural. Unlike most other body-care products, it can be used in its natural form without adulteration by harsh chemicals and other additives. For this reason, it has been used for many years as a body cream and lotion.

Skin Elasticity Test

How youthful is your skin? As we age, our skin loses its elasticity, becoming leathery and wrinkled. This is the result of free-radical destruction and is a sign of degeneration and loss of function. Significant changes in the skin become evident at about age 45. The following skin test indicates approximately how old functionally the skin has become as a result of free-radical deterioration. Take this test and see how your skin rates as compared with the age groups listed. Test to see if your skin is functionally younger or older than your biological age.

For this test, pinch the skin on the back of your hand with the thumb and forefinger and hold it for five seconds. Let go and time how long it takes for the skin to completely flatten back out. The shorter the time, the younger the functional age of the skin. Compare your results to the table.

TIME (SECONDS)	FUNCTIONAL AGE (YEARS)
1–2	under 30
3–4	30–44
5–9	45–50
10–15	60
35–55	70
56 or more	over 70

How did you fare? Did your skin test older than your true age, or were you right on target? If you want to prevent further degeneration and perhaps even regain some youthfulness in your skin, the best thing you can do is use coconut oil in place of other creams and lotions. I'm in my fifties and when I perform this test, my skin bounces back within 1–2 seconds—just as you would expect from a 20-year-old.

KEEPING YOUR SKIN SMOOTH AND AGELESS

We use hand and body lotions to soften the skin and make it look younger. Many lotions, however, actually promote dry skin. Commercial creams are predominantly water. Their moisture is quickly absorbed into dry, wrinkled skin. As the water enters the skin, it expands the tissues, like filling a balloon with water, so that wrinkles fade away and skin feels smoother. But this is only temporary. As soon as the water evaporates or is carried away by the bloodstream, the dry, wrinkled skin returns. Ordinary body-care products cannot permanently cure dry, wrinkled skin. Most lotions contain some type of highly processed vegetable oils that are devoid of all the natural, protective antioxidants that are so important to skin care.

Oils have a pronounced effect on all the tissues of the body, especially the connective tissues. Connective tissue is the most abundant and widely distributed tissue in the body; it is found in the skin, the muscles, the bones, the nerves, and all the internal organs. Connective tissue consists of strong fibers that form the matrix, or supporting framework, for all body tissues. In other words, it holds everything together. Without connective fibers, we would become a shapeless mass of tissue. They give the skin strength and elasticity. When we are young and healthy the skin is smooth, elastic, and supple. As we age these fibers are continually breaking down because of free-radical attack, causing them to sag and wrinkle. The once young, soft, and smooth skin turns dry and leathery.

Once a free-radical reaction is started, it can cause a chain reaction that produces more free radicals, which ultimately damages thousands of molecules. The only way our body has to fight them is with antioxidants. When a free radical comes into contact with an antioxidant, the chain reaction is stopped. For this reason, it's good to have plenty of antioxidants available in our cells and tissues to protect us. The number of antioxidants we have in our tissues is determined to a large extent by the nutrients in our diet.

Free-radical reactions occur in the body constantly, and they are an unavoidable result of living and breathing. However, some people experience more free-radical damage than others. The reason is that there are many environmental factors that increase the number of free-radical reactions we are subjected to. For example, a diet low in antioxidant nutrients (vitamins A, C, and E, for example) will lower the amount of antioxidants our cells have available to protect themselves. Cigarette smoke and pollution readily create free radicals. Radiation, including ultraviolet light, can stimulate free-radical generation. Chemicals such as pesticides and food additives also increase free-radical activity. One substance that is commonly used in our food, and even in body-care products, and that leads to a great deal of free radicals is oxidized vegetable oil.

Conventional processing strips polyunsaturated oils from the natural antioxidants that protect them. Without these antioxidants, they are highly prone to free-radical generation, both inside and outside of the body. When we eat processed oils, our body has to use antioxidants to fight off the free radicals contained in the oil, resulting in a deficiency in vitamin E and other antioxidants. When we put these types of oils on our skin they also create free radicals, causing permanent damage to connective tissues. This is why you should be very careful about the types of oils you use on your skin. If you use a lotion or cream containing this type of oil you are, in effect, causing your skin to age faster. The lotion may bring temporary improvement but accelerate aging of the skin and even promote skin cancer.

One of the classic signs of old age is the appearance of brown, frecklelike spots on the skin. This pigment is called *lipofuscin*. It is also known as aging spots or liver spots. It is a sign of free-radical deterioration of the lipids (fats) in our skin, thus the name lipofuscin. Oxidation of polyunsaturated fats and protein by free-radical activity in the skin is recognized as the major cause of liver spots. Liver spots don't ordinarily hurt or show any signs of discomfort. If we couldn't see them we wouldn't even know they were there. But they do affect our health and our appearance.

While liver spots are clearly seen on the skin, they also form in other tissues throughout the body—intestines, lungs, kidney, brain, and so on. They represent areas that are damaged by free-radical reactions. The more you have on your skin, the more you have inside your body, and the more damage or "aging" your tissues have undergone. To some degree you can judge the damage free radicals have done to the inside of your body by the size and number of liver spots on your skin. The more you have and the bigger they are, the more free-radical damage has occurred. All the tissues affected are damaged to some degree. If this occurs in your intestine, it can affect the organ's ability to digest and absorb nutrients. In the brain it will affect mental ability. Likewise, free radicals break down connective tissues, causing sagging and loss of function of the skin. And the same thing happens to the internal organs; they sag and become deformed. The skin acts as a window by which we can see inside the body. What we look like on the outside reflects, to a large part, what is happening on the inside.

Because cells cannot dispose of the lipofuscin pigment, it gradually accumulates within many cells of the body as we age. Once lipofuscin pigment develops, it tends to stick around for life, but you can prevent further oxidation and perhaps even reduce the spots you already have by using the right kind of oils in your diet and on your skin.

HEALING YOUR SKIN WITH COCONUT OIL

The ideal lotion is one that not only softens the skin but also protects it against damage, promotes healing, and gives it a more youthful, healthy appearance. Pure coconut oil is the best natural skin lotion available. It prevents free-radical formation and the damage it causes. It can help prevent the skin from developing liver spots and other blemishes caused by aging and overexposure to sunlight. It helps to keep connective tissues strong and supple so that the skin doesn't sag and wrinkle. In some cases it can even restore damaged or diseased skin. I've seen precancerous lesions completely disappear with the daily use of coconut oil.

The Polynesians, who traditionally wear very little clothing, have for generations been exposed to the hot blistering sun, yet have beautiful healthy skin without blemishes and without cancer. The reason is they eat coconuts and use the oil on their bodies as a lotion. The oil is absorbed into the skin and into the cell structure of the connective tissues, limiting the damage excessive sun exposure can cause. Their skin remains undamaged even when exposed to long hours in the hot sun.

The difference between coconut oil and other creams and lotions is that the latter are made to bring immediate, temporary relief. Coconut oil, on the other hand, not only brings quick relief but also aids in the healing and repairing process. Most lotions do the skin no lasting benefit, and many actually accelerate the aging process. Why take the risk of permanently damaging the skin when you can easily use coconut oil to help bring back its youthful appearance?

Coconut oil can make your skin look more youthful. The surface of the skin consists of a layer of dead cells. As these dead cells fall off, new cells take their place. As we age, this process slows down, and dead cells tend to accumulate, giving the skin a rough, flaky texture. Coconut oil aids in removing dead cells on the outer surface of the skin, making the skin smoother, enabling it to reflect light more evenly, creating a healthier, more youthful appearance. The skin "shines" because light reflects better off evenly textured skin.

The removal of excessive dead skin and the strengthening of underlying tissues are two of the key advantages to using coconut oil as a skin lotion. Sometimes even young people can be troubled with chapped or excessively dry skin, producing an abnormally thick and often irritating layer of dead cells. Coconut oil not only provides immediate relief but often brings lasting improvement as well. People with a variety of skin problems have experienced remarkable results from using coconut oil. Many people who have tried it won't use anything else.

When using coconut oil as a lotion, it is best to apply a small amount and reapply it as often as necessary. When first applied it may seem like you're spreading a very oily substance on your skin, but because it is quickly absorbed, it doesn't leave a layer of greasy film the way many commercial lotions and oils do. If you apply too much oil all at once, the skin becomes saturated and will not absorb it all. This will leave a greasy film. People with extremely dry skin need to reapply the oil often when they first start using it. Some people with this problem desire the greasiness common with many lotions to soften extremely dry or hardened skin. At first they don't think the coconut oil does enough because it is absorbed so quickly. With coconut oil you will need to reapply the oil more often when the skin is very dry. The real benefit of

> "For a number of years I had been troubled occasionally with severely dry, cracked skin on my hands. It would come without warning and persist for a couple of months, then gradually get better. Nothing I did seemed to help. The last time it appeared was the most severe. At times the skin would be so dry it would crack and bleed. My wife avoided holding my hand because she said it felt like sandpaper. And it did!
>
> "I tried a variety of creams and lotions without success. The condition persisted for over a year, much longer than it ever had before. I then learned about coconut oil and how good it is for the skin. I bought some coconut oil and began applying it to my hands. Immediately I noticed a difference. I hated to use lotions because they often left a greasy or sticky film on my hands, but coconut oil soaked into the skin without that feeling. Best of all, within a couple of weeks my rough, dry skin went away—permanently. My hands are now very smooth and soft. When I'm out with my wife, she gladly takes hold of my hand, just as she used to do. Coconut oil is without reservation the best skin care product I have ever used."
>
> —*Tom M.*

coconut oil will come with repeated use over time. While other lotions temporarily soften dry skin, they won't heal it. Coconut oil will gradually soften the skin, removing dead layers, and encourage the growth of new, healthier tissue.

If dryness and cracking are severe, I recommend applying a liberal amount of coconut oil to the affected area and then wrapping it loosely in plastic (so it doesn't drip all over the place) before going to sleep at night. In the morning remove the plastic and wash off the excess oil. Do this every night until the condition improves. A waterproof, self-adhesive bandage made by 3M, called Tegaderm, makes an excellent wrapping for this purpose.

PROTECTING THE SKIN FROM GERMS

Whether it is applied topically or taken internally, coconut oil helps to keep skin young, healthy, and free of disease. When coconut oil is consumed in the diet and, to some extent, when it is applied directly, antiseptic fatty acids help to prevent fungal and bacterial infections in the skin. The Polynesians who use it regularly are rarely troubled by skin infections or acne.

Our skin acts as a protective covering, shielding us from harm much like a suit of flexible armor. It provides a protective barrier between us and literally millions of disease-causing germs that we come into contact with each day. If it were not for our skin, we could not survive; even organisms that are ordinarily harmless would become deadly.

The only way to gain entry into the body, other than through the natural openings such as the nose and mouth, is by penetrating the skin. When the skin's defenses break down, infections can result. Acne, ringworm, herpes, boils, athlete's foot, and warts are just some of the infectious conditions that can affect the skin and body.

Our skin is more than simply a covering. If that was all it was, we would literally be covered with disease-causing germs just waiting for an opportunity to gain entry into the body. The slightest cut, even a tiny scratch, would allow a multitude of these troublemakers into the body, causing disease and perhaps death. Fortunately, the skin provides not only a physical barrier but a chemical one as well. The chemical environment on the surface of healthy skin is inhospitable to most harmful germs. As a consequence, organisms that cause disease are few in number. Most cuts do not end up becoming infected because the skin is relatively free from harmful germs. However, if a wound is made by an object such as a dirty nail that is covered in dangerous microorganisms, they bypass the skin's physical and chemical barriers, and infection often results.

The biggest chemical barrier to infectious organisms is the acid layer on the skin. Healthy skin has a pH of about 5, making it slightly acidic. Our sweat (containing uric and lactic acids) and body oils promote this acidic environment. For this reason, sweat and oil do us good. Harmless bacteria that can tolerate the acid live on the skin, but troublesome bacteria can't thrive, and their numbers are few.

The oil our bodies produce, called sebum, is secreted by oil glands (sebaceous glands) that are located at the root of every hair as well as in other places. This oil is very important to skin health. It softens and lubricates the skin and hair and prevents the skin from drying and cracking. Sebum also contains medium-chain fatty acids, in the form of medium-chain triglycerides, that can be released to fight harmful germs.

Our skin is home to many tiny organisms, most of which are harmless; some are even beneficial. Lipophilic bacteria are essential to the healthy environment on our skin. They feed on the sebum, breaking down the triglycerides—three fatty acids joined by a glycerol molecule. (Sebum, as well as all dietary fats [e.g. coconut oil, corn oil, soybean oil, etc.], is composed primarily of triglycerides.) These bacteria feed on the glycerol molecule that holds the fatty acids together. When the glycerol is removed, the fatty acids are freed and become independent of one another: this is what is called a free fatty acid.

Medium-chain fatty acids bound together as triglycerides have no antimicrobial properties, but when broken down into free fatty acids, they become powerful antimicrobials that can kill disease-causing bacteria, viruses, and fungi. Thus the combination of the skin's pH and these MCFAs provide a protective chemical layer on the skin that prevents infection from these microorganisms.

Most, if not all, mammals utilize the antimicrobial property of medium-chain fatty acids to protect themselves from infection. As in humans, these fatty acids make up a part of the oil excreted by the skin. In the wild, animals are left to nature and instinct to heal from injury. Bites and scratches are common occurrences, especially from encounters with predators. Wounds from these animals can often cause infection in a victim that is lucky enough to escape with its life. Instinctively, injured animals will lick the wound to clean it out and to spread body oils into the injured tissue. These oils disinfect the wound, thus protecting the animal from infection. Likewise, when we cut a finger we instinctively put the injured part of the finger in our mouths.

The saliva also helps to increase the amount of MCFAs on the skin. Saliva contains an enzyme called lingual lipase, which begins the process of breaking fats down into individual fatty acids. This enzyme readily breaks down the medium-chain triglycerides in dietary fats and body oils (sebum) into free medium-chain fatty acids. Fats and oils made of long-chain fatty acids, as most all dietary fats are, need the addition of gastric and pancreatic enzymes to break them all the way down to individual fatty acids.

Animals often cleanse themselves by licking their fur, coating it with salivary enzymes that can convert body oils into protective free MCFAs. Licking a wound also mixes saliva with the oils on the skin and hair, producing more medium-chain fatty acids that can help fight infection. Some animals seem to produce more of these protective fatty acids than others. The porcupine is one of these. The porcupine's quills make an intimidating weapon; unfortunately, these critters can accidentally impale themselves or other porcupines. Dr. Uldis Roze, a biology professor at Queens College in New York, speculates that the high amount of protective fatty acids is a defense against self-inflicted wounds (Nochan, 1994). Dr. Roze found out about the antimicrobial properties of fatty acids on porcupine quills the hard way. His research involves tracking porcupines, capturing them, and attaching radio collars. One day he followed a porcupine up a tree and in his attempt to capture it took a quill in his upper arm. Unable to remove the quill, he waited for it to work itself out. A few days later when the quill came through, Dr. Roze was surprised that the deep puncture wound remained free from infection. He reasoned that a wood splinter traveling the same path would almost certainly have caused a serious infection. Roze theorized that the oil on the quill contained antibiotic properties that protected him. This theory was verified when the oil was analyzed and tested. The medium-chain fatty acids in the oil proved to be the secret. His studies showed that these fatty acids could kill several types of bacteria that are often treated by penicillin, including streptococcus and staphylococcus.

He approached the pharmaceutical industry in an attempt to interest them in producing an antibiotic ointment or medication using these fatty acids. He was turned down because medium-chain fatty acids are readily available, natural substances and therefore could not be protected by a patent.

We all have this protection on our skin to various degrees. Primarily because of the action of friendly bacteria, the oil on the surface of your skin and hair is composed of between 40 to 60 percent free fatty acids, among them the medium-chain fatty acids that have antimicrobial properties. They provide the protective layer on the skin that kills harmful germs.

Adults produce more sebum than children and therefore have a greater degree of protection from skin infections. The antimicrobial effects of MCFAs in sebum have been observed at least as far back as the 1940s. At the time it was noted that children suffering with scalp ringworm (a skin fungus) were cured spontaneously when sebum secretion increased as they reached puberty.

Medium-chain fatty acids similar to those in sebum are found abundantly in coconut oil. The fatty acids in coconut oil, like all other dietary oils, are joined together as triglycerides. Triglycerides, as such, have no antimicrobial properties, even when they are made of MCFAs. However, when we eat medium-chain triglycerides, our bodies convert them into monoglycerides and free fatty acids, which do have antimicrobial properties.

When coconut oil, which is made of triglycerides, is put on the skin, it doesn't have any immediate antimicrobial action. However, the bacteria that are always present on the skin turn these triglycerides into free fatty acids, just as they do with sebum. The result is an increase in the number of antimicrobial fatty acids on the skin and protection from infection. The free fatty acids also help to contribute to the acidic environment on the skin, which repels disease-causing germs. After all, fatty acids are acidic and therefore support the acid layer on the skin.

When bathing or showering, soap washes the protective layer of oil and acid off our skin. Often afterward the skin becomes tight and dry. Adding moisturizers helps the skin feel better, but it does not replace the acid or the protective MCFAs that were removed. Your skin is vulnerable to infection at this time. You would think that your body would be clean and germ free after a bath. But germs are everywhere, floating in the air, on our clothes and everything we touch. Many germs survive washing by hiding in cracks and folds of the skin. Before long your skin is again teaming with microscopic life, both good and bad. Until sweat and oils return to reestablish the body's chemical barrier, your skin is vulnerable to infection. If you have a cut or cracked skin, this can allow streptococcus, staphylococcus, and other harmful germs entry into the body. By using a coconut or palm kernel oil–based lotion, you can quickly help reestablish the skin's natural antimicrobial

"It's only been about three months since I began using coconut oil. My skin is like a newborn babe's. My face is lovely and rosy. The bottoms of my feet are like a teenager's (I don't rub it in, I merely ingest it). For the first time in 53-plus years I am WARM as long as I use the coconut oil. And I've lost 11 pounds. My hair is beautiful! As far as I'm concerned virgin coconut oil is my miracle food."

—*Linda P.*

and acid barrier. If you are troubled with skin infections or want to avoid infections, it would be to your benefit to use coconut oil after every bath.

HAIR CARE

What coconut oil does for the skin it can also do for the hair. It makes a great hair conditioner. The noted New York hair stylist Amanda George gives credit to coconut oil for her luxurious hair. "I massage two teaspoons of warm coconut oil into my hair before bed, then wash it out in the morning," says Amanda. The result is hair that is soft and shimmering. To warm the oil you can place the bottle in warm water or hold it briefly under hot running tap water.

Beauticians who are familiar with coconut oil swear by it. They claim that it can be just as effective for conditioning hair as a $40 or $50 salon treatment—at only a fraction of the cost. And you can do it yourself at home.

A little oil (a couple of teaspoons) can be applied at night and washed out in the morning, or you can use a little more and thoroughly soak the hair for an hour or two before washing. Some people prefer to put the oil on, cover the head with a shower cap, and then take a long relaxing bath. After about an hour the oil is washed off. This process can be repeated every few days.

If you take a long warm bath make sure to apply coconut oil on your skin to replace the natural oils that have been washed off. In fact, any time you use soap you are removing your body's protective layer of oil and changing the pH of your skin. Applying coconut oil will help reestablish a healthy skin environment.

Another advantage of using coconut oil as a hair conditioner is that it will help control dandruff. I found this out for myself. I've been plagued with dandruff since I was a teenager. The only thing that could control it was to use medicated shampoos, which I did for many years. Whenever I tried switching to a nonmedicated shampoo, the dandruff came right back within a few days. As I learned more about the harsh chemicals used in many body-care products, I decided I didn't want to use medicated shampoos anymore. I started to use more natural herbal soaps and shampoos. As before, the dandruff came roaring back in full force. I tried everything natural I could find in an attempt to control it. Nothing seemed to work. I eventually put some coconut oil in my hair, as just described, and washed it out several hours later. The result was phenomenal. After a single application all the dandruff was gone. I couldn't believe it was that easy. Nothing except medicated shampoos had worked this well before. I now have a natural product that has not only cleared up my dandruff but is good for my hair and scalp as well. Coconut oil is now a regular part of my personal care regimen.

NATURE'S MIRACLE HEALING SALVE

While the antimicrobial power of MCFAs in coconut oil has been experimentally tested in the laboratory, used in biology, and seen in everyday life, there is another side to the healing power of coconut oil when applied topically. This was shown to me by accident.

I experienced the healing power of coconut oil in an unusual way. I was unloading a carload of cement blocks. If you've ever worked with cement blocks you know they are heavy. When I went to set one down, I accidentally pinched a piece of the flesh of my hand between two of the blocks. The pain was intense but hardly life-threatening, so I continued on with the task. Immediately a dark red blood blister started to form. When I finished unloading the blocks, I washed my hands and applied some coconut oil, simply as a moisturizer, and thought nothing more of it.

A few hours later I looked at the blister, and it had shrunk from the size of a split pea to that of a pinhead. I was amazed. I'd never seen a blood blister fade away that quickly. Usually they take a week or two to heal. Since I hadn't done anything except put coconut oil on it, my first thought was perhaps the oil was somehow involved in the rapid healing. I immediately dismissed the idea as silly and ignored it. I knew coconut oil was good when eaten, but to speed the healing of an injury on the skin seemed too remarkable.

Later I began to see similar miracles in others who had used the oil topically. For example, one of my clients told me he had a flare-up with hemorrhoids that were causing him a great deal of pain and discomfort. He tried various creams, but they didn't help. He had just purchased a jar of coconut oil and thought he might try that. So he began applying the oil to the affected area, and to his joy and amazement it relieved the irritation. By the next day the swelling was also gone.

In another case a man had been troubled with psoriasis on his face and chest, essentially all his adult life. He tried every cream, ointment, and salve that came along and nothing worked. Every few days the condition would flare up, the skin would become dry and scaly, and sometimes it would get so bad it would crack and bleed. It affected his forehead, eyebrows, nose, cheeks, chin, and chest. As he got older the condition worsened to the point that inflammation and peeling became a constant nuisance. He'd gone to several doctors, and they told him there was nothing they could do to cure the problem and that he might get some temporary relief using a prescription cream. The cream provided only minor temporary relief. Because he didn't get the help he sought from medical doctors, he turned to alternative therapies and began to focus on solving his problem through diet. He cut out convenience foods, reducing sugar and vegetable oil consumption. Eventually he replaced most of the oils in his diet with coconut oil. The condition gradually improved but still didn't go away. While the severity of the psoriasis was much reduced, the inflammation and scaling persisted. One day when the inflammation was flaring up he applied a little coconut oil to see what that would do. It worked! He did it again the next day and the next. Within just a few days the skin on his face, which had once been almost constantly dry and leathery, now became soft and smooth. No inflammation and no scaling. He says it's the best his skin has looked in over 20 years!

One lady told me, "I like using coconut oil on my face. It keeps my skin moist without making it greasy." She compared it to the medicated cream Retin-A that has been touted by some as a wonder drug. "I used to use Retin-A to prevent pimples," she told me, "but since I've been using coconut oil I haven't needed it. It works just as well as Retin-A." Retin-A is a medicated cream prescribed by doctors to prevent acne and improve skin texture. While it provides some benefits, it also causes undesirable side effects, the worst of which is making the skin hypersensitive to sunlight, which increases the potential for sunburn and skin cancer. This is why it is only available by prescription from a medical doctor.

Coconut oil is the perfect medium for almost any herbal salve. One such salve, called GOOT (garlic oil ointment), consists of crushed raw garlic in coconut oil. It's an ointment you can make yourself and is effective against skin infections. Mark Konlee, the editor of *Positive Health News*, says, "I have never ceased to be amazed at what this ointment can accomplish. Last fall, I met 'Dan,' a local resident who told me he had a bad case of plantar warts and athlete's foot. When he showed me the soles of his feet, it was the worst-looking set of feet I have ever observed."

Mark made some GOOT, put it in a small jar, and gave it to Dan. He told him to keep the bottle in the refrigerator (shelf life of about 30 days) and put a little on his feet every day. Two weeks later he met Dan again. "He took off his socks to show me what looked like a magical transformation—both the fungal infection and the plantar warts were completely gone. He had what looked like a brand new set of feet, totally normal in color and appearance." Dan reported, "After about 10 days, the plantar warts just peeled off."

Many people claim that, when applied to the skin, coconut oil helps protect them from sunburn and consequently from problems related to overexposure to ultraviolet light, such as the development of skin cancer and aging spots. Premature wrinkling and dry skin can also be a consequence of too much sun. Coconut oil helps protect the skin from the damaging rays of the sun while allowing the body to gradually adapt so it can withstand greater and greater amounts of exposure. Unlike sunscreen, coconut oil doesn't necessarily block UV light but enables the body to adjust naturally to sun exposure, naturally increasing the body's tolerance level over time. Because of different skin types, everybody's level of tolerance is different, so each person needs to experiment, getting a little more sun each day until he or she reaches a level of exposure that feels comfortable. Traditionally the Polynesians wore very little clothing and exposed themselves to the hot tropical sun nearly all day long. This was especially true when they traveled long distances over open oceans for days or weeks at a time. Coconut oil supplied them with the protection they needed. For this reason, coconut oil is a common ingredient in many commercial sunscreen and suntan lotions.

Why is coconut oil able to stimulate healing and repair? I think it is, in part, because of the metabolic effect MCFAs have on the cells. Cellular activity, including healing of injuries, is regulated by the metabolism. When metabolic rate is high, cellular activity is accelerated, and processes such as healing damaged tissues, removing toxins, fighting

---

"I started taking coconut oil internally for its many benefits five weeks ago. Immediately I noticed a consistently higher energy level, as well as a drastic decrease in my cravings for junk food. I also began using the coconut oil on my face and body, but I never expected to watch years' worth of keloid scars from injuries, surgeries, and acne start vanishing before my eyes. The deep pink color is fading quickly, the thick overgrowth of skin is shrinking, and the itching has completely disappeared. Scars were an area of my life that I had truly given up on, as all the treatments I had tried in the past failed miserably. I'm so thankful to be regaining the smooth, unblemished skin I had as a teenager."

—*Alicia Voorhies, RN*

germs, replacing damaged or diseased cells with healthy new ones, and such are all performed at a heightened rate of activity. Therefore, the healing process is accelerated; MCFAs provide a quick source of energy to the cells, boosting their metabolic level and healing capacity.

One of the things that has impressed me most about the topical use of coconut oil is its ability to reduce inflammation. I've seen it relieve chronic skin inflammation within days. At first this effect was a surprise to me, for at the time I had not found any reference in the scientific literature to coconut oil's effect on inflammation. With further searching I did locate a study that demonstrated that coconut oil does indeed have an anti-inflammatory effect. In a study reported by Dr. S. Sadeghi and others, coconut oil reduced proinflammatory chemicals in the body. The researchers suggested that coconut oil might be useful in therapies involving a number of acute and chronic inflammatory diseases. This would help explain my observation that psoriasis and other inflammatory skin conditions seem to improve with the application of coconut oil. I have found, however, that it doesn't work in all cases. If inflammation is severe, coconut oil alone isn't enough to eliminate it. But for mild cases it has worked well.

It is interesting to note that when it is taken internally, the healing characteristics coconut oil exhibits on the skin are also in effect inside the body. Conditions associated with inflammation (especially within the gastrointestinal tract), such as colitis, ulcers, hepatitis, and hemorrhoids, may be relieved by this natural, harmless oil. It may also relieve inflammation in other parts of the body, as has been seen in multiple sclerosis, arthritis, lupus, and the inflammation in the arteries (phlebitis) that can lead to hardening of the arteries and heart disease.

Some of these inflammatory conditions are caused by infections from microorganisms. Most ulcers are caused by bacteria. Inflamed arteries and heart disease can be caused by viruses and bacteria. Hepatitis is usually caused by viral infections in the liver. Coconut oil's antimicrobial effects can eliminate the offending organisms and relieve the inflammation and pain they cause.

It appears that coconut oil, whether used inside or outside the body, provides numerous health benefits. Coconut is truly one of nature's miracle foods. It is no wonder that the early European explorers who visited the Pacific Islands were greatly impressed by the natives' excellent health and physical condition.

7

COCONUT OIL AS FOOD AND AS MEDICINE

Let me take you to the jungles of northern Brazil, far from civilization. Imagine yourself as a modern-day explorer venturing into the Amazon rain forest fighting pesky mosquitoes and wading through knee-deep swamps. One morning you wake up sweating like an ice cube in the hot July sun. A fever rages out of control, interspersed with brief periods of icy chills. Every muscle in your body feels like it's twisted into knots; the strain has sapped your strength, and you lie exhausted, almost too weak to move. With no modern medicine or doctors to help, you seek assistance from the natives. Your health, perhaps even your life, depends on the skill of the tribal medicine man. His treatment consists of a porridge made from coconut. You're fed this meal every day. Under the watchful care of the medicine man, you gradually regain your strength, and soon you're well enough to go on your way.

This story is not beyond belief. The natives of South and Central America regard coconut as both a food and a medicine. It helps to keep them healthy in a climate infested with malaria, yellow fever, and other tropical diseases. If you go along the coasts of Somalia and Ethiopia in Africa, the locals will give you palm kernel oil if you are sick—a traditional remedy used for almost all ills. Whether you are on an island in

Disease Prevention and Treatment Uses for Coconut Oil

Research and clinical observation have shown that medium-chain fatty acids, like those found in coconut oil, may help prevent and treat a wide range of diseases. Coconut oil can help:

- Prevent heart disease, high blood pressure, atherosclerosis, and stroke
- Prevent diabetes and relieve the symptoms and health risks associated with the disease
- Support the development of strong bones and teeth
- Protect against osteoporosis
- Promote loss of excess weight
- Kill viruses that cause mononucleosis, influenza, hepatitis C, measles, herpes, AIDS, and other illnesses
- Reduce symptoms associated with pancreatitis
- Reduce severity of problems associated with malabsorption syndrome and cystic fibrosis
- Relieve symptoms of gallbladder disease
- Relieve symptoms associated with Crohn's disease, ulcerative colitis, and stomach ulcers
- Relieve pain and irritation caused by hemorrhoids
- Reduce chronic inflammation
- Protect the body from breast, colon, and other cancers
- Prevent periodontal disease and tooth decay
- Prevent premature aging and degenerative disease
- Relieve symptoms associated with chronic fatigue syndrome
- Relieve symptoms associated with benign prostatic hyperplasia (prostate enlargement)
- Reduce epileptic seizures
- Protect against kidney disease and bladder infections
- Prevent liver disease

- Kill bacteria that cause pneumonia, earache, throat infections, dental cavities, food poisoning, urinary tract infections, meningitis, gonorrhea, and dozens of other diseases
- Kill fungi and yeast that cause candida, jock itch, ringworm, athlete's foot, thrush, diaper rash, and other infections
- Expel or kill tapeworms, lice, giardia, and other parasites
- Ward off skin infections
- Reduce symptoms associated with psoriasis, eczema, and dermatitis
- Relieve dryness and flaking
- Prevent damaging effects of UV radiation from the sun such as wrinkles, sagging skin, and age spots
- Control dandruff

the Caribbean, an atoll in the Pacific Ocean, or the coast of Southeast Asia or India, it is likely that the native people would give you coconut in some form as part of your treatment. Wherever the coconut palm grows, the people have learned of its value as a source of food and as a medicine. This is why it is hailed as the Tree of Life.

Coconut and coconut oil are used in many traditional forms of medicine. The most well known of these is the Ayurvedic medicine of India. Here coconut products enjoy a place of importance and are essential components of some of the medicinal preparations. Coconut oil is recognized for its healing properties in both Ayurvedic and Indian folkloric medicine to treat a variety of conditions such as burns, wounds, ulcers, skin fungus, lice, kidney stones, and choleraic dysentery.

Modern medical science is just now beginning to unlock the healing secrets of coconut oil. Research is showing that coconut oil has many practical applications as a medicine. At this point you have learned how coconut oil can help protect against heart disease. The MCFAs in coconut oil have a powerful antimicrobial effect that can kill a wide variety of infectious organisms, even the supergerms that are resistant to drugs. Coconut oil has proved to be a superfood that is easily digested and utilized to nourish the body. Medical research and clinical experience is continually uncovering additional uses for this miracle oil.

DIGESTIVE AND NUTRIENT ABSORPTION DISORDERS

For at least five decades researchers have recognized that MCFAs are digested differently from other fats. This difference has had important applications in the treatment of many digestive and metabolic health conditions, and during that time MCFAs have been routinely used in hospital and baby formulas.

The digestive health advantages of medium-chain fatty acids over long-chain fatty acids are due to the differences in the way our bodies metabolize these fats. Because the MCFA molecules are smaller, they require less energy and fewer enzymes to break them down for digestion. They are digested and absorbed quickly and with minimal effort.

The MCFAs are broken down almost immediately by enzymes in the saliva and gastric juices so that pancreatic fat-digesting enzymes are not even essential. Therefore, there is less strain on the pancreas and digestive system. This has important implications for patients who suffer from digestive and metabolic problems. Premature and ill infants especially, whose digestive organs are underdeveloped, are able to absorb MCFAs with relative ease, while other fats pass through their systems pretty much undigested. People who suffer from malabsorption problems such as cystic fibrosis and have difficulty digesting or absorbing fats and fat-soluble vitamins benefit greatly from MCFAs. They can also be important for people suffering from diabetes, obesity, gallbladder disease, pancreatitis, Crohn's disease, pancreatic insufficiency, and some forms of cancer.

As we get older, our bodies don't function as well as they did in earlier years. The pancreas doesn't make as many digestive enzymes; our intestines don't absorb nutrients as well; the whole process of digestion and elimination moves at a lower rate of efficiency. As a result, older people often suffer from vitamin and mineral deficiencies. Because MCFAs are easy to digest and improve vitamin and mineral absorption, they should be included in the meals of older people. This is easy to do if the meals are prepared with coconut oil.

Unlike other fatty acids, MCFAs are absorbed directly from the intestines into the portal vein and sent straight to the liver, where they are, for the most part, burned as fuel, much like a carbohydrate. In this respect they act more like carbohydrates than like fats.

Other fats require pancreatic enzymes to break them into smaller units. They are then absorbed into the intestinal wall and packaged into bundles of fat (lipid) and protein called lipoproteins. These lipoproteins are carried by the lymphatic system, bypassing the liver, and then dumped into the bloodstream, where they are circulated throughout the body. As they circulate in the blood, their fatty components are distributed to all the tissues of the body. The lipoproteins get smaller and smaller, until there is little left of them. At this time they are picked up by the liver, broken apart, and used to produce energy or, if needed, repackaged into other lipoproteins and sent back into the bloodstream to be distributed throughout the body. Cholesterol, saturated fat, monounsaturated fat, and polyunsaturated fat are all packaged together into lipoproteins and carried throughout the body in this way. In contrast, MCFAs are not packaged into lipoproteins in the intestinal tract but go straight to the liver, where they are converted into energy. Ordinarily they are not stored to any significant degree as body fat. While MCFAs produce energy, other dietary fats produce body fat.

Cells get all the energy they need to carry on their metabolic functions from glucose and fatty acids. Long-chain fatty acids, as well as glucose, require the hormone insulin to transport them through the cell wall. Without insulin, glucose and LCFAs could not enter the cells. This is of major concern for people who are insulin resistant, such as those with Type II diabetes. If the cells cannot get enough glucose or fatty acids, they literally starve to death. Medium-chain fatty acids have an advantage in that they do not require insulin to enter the cells. They can easily penetrate the cell wall without it.

Inside all of our cells are organelles called mitochondria. The energy needed by cells to carry on their functions is generated by the mitochondria. Mitochondria are encased in two membranous sacs, which normally require special enzymes to transport nutrients through them. MCFAs are unique in that they can easily permeate both membranes of the mitochondria without the need of enzymes and thus provide the cell with a quick and efficient source of energy. Long-chain fatty acids demand special enzymes to pull them through the double membrane, and this energy production process is much slower and taxing on enzyme reserves.

Because of these advantages, coconut oil has been a lifesaver for many people, particularly the very young and the very old. It is used medicinally in special food preparations for those who suffer digestive disorders and have trouble digesting fats. For the same reason, it is also used in infant formula and for the treatment of malnutrition. Since it is rapidly absorbed, it can deliver quick nourishment without putting excessive strain on the digestive and enzyme systems and can help conserve the energy that would normally be expended in digesting other fats.

NOURISHMENT FOR NEWBORN BABIES

Among all the foods in nature there is one that stands head and shoulders above all the rest. That food is mother's milk. Milk was designed by nature to supply all the nutrients a baby needs for the first year or so of life. It contains a perfect blend of vitamins, minerals, proteins, and fats for optimal growth and development. Without question, breast milk is one of the wonders of nature. Children who are breast-fed not only take in important nutrients from the milk but also receive antibodies and other substances necessary to protect them against childhood illnesses, such as ear infections, later in life. Breast-fed children have better teeth and jaw formation, are less prone to allergies, have better digestive function, and are better able to fight off infectious disease. Research suggests that breast-fed children may even develop higher intelligence. Recognizing the superiority of nature, scientists have attempted to make baby formula match mother's milk as closely as possible.

An important component of breast milk is medium-chain fatty acids, principally lauric acid. Lauric acid is also the primary saturated fatty acid found in coconut oil. The medium-chain fatty acids in breast milk improve nutrient absorption, aid digestive function, help regulate blood sugar levels, and protect the baby from harmful microorganisms. The baby's immature immune system is supported by the antibacterial, antiviral, antifungal, and antiparasitic properties of these vital fatty acids. In fact, without these unique saturated fats, the baby would probably not survive long. It would become malnourished and highly susceptible to a myriad of infectious diseases.

Milk that is rich in MCFAs is vital for the healthy growth and development of the child. In a recent study, vegetable oil or coconut oil was added to the formula of 46 very-low-birthweight babies to see if supplementation was capable of enhancing their weight gain. The group with the coconut oil gained weight quicker. The weight gain was due to physical growth, not fat storage. The babies gained more weight and grew better with the coconut oil because their bodies were able to digest it easily. The vegetable oils, to a great extent, passed through their digestive tracts undigested and thus deprived them of nutrients they needed for proper development. The MCFAs not only allow infants to absorb needed fats but also improve the absorption of fat-soluble vitamins, minerals, and protein.

MCFAs are added to most, if not all, baby formulas. At one time formula manufacturers used pure coconut or palm kernel oils, and some brands still do, but MCT oil is used in many formulas. This oil is a product of industry that contains 75 percent caprylic acid and 25 percent capric acid, with little or no lauric acid—the most important antimicrobial MCFA. Lauric acid is also the most abundant MCFA found naturally in mother's milk. The ratio of lauric acid to other MCFAs in coconut oil is similar to that in mother's milk. The reason MCT oil is used in place of the more expensive coconut oil has to do with economics rather than health concerns. Don't get me wrong, caprylic and capric acids are good, but not as good as lauric acid, and not as good as a combination of all three, as nature intended.

Just as the fatty acid content and quality of formula can be altered, so can human breast milk. Breast milk is, without question, the best choice of food for babies. Not all breast milk is the same, however. The quality of the milk is influenced by the mother's health and diet. Breast milk is made from the nutrients the mother consumes. If she doesn't eat the right amount of nutrients, her body will pull them out of her own tissues. If the mother is deficient in these vital nutrients herself, then the milk she produces will also be deficient. Similarly, if she eats foods containing toxins (such as trans fatty acids) her milk may contain them as well. Eating wisely is very important for pregnant and nursing women and their babies.

Human milk fat has a unique fatty acid composition of 45–50 percent saturated fat, 35 percent monounsaturated fat, and 15–20 percent polyunsaturated fat. A significant portion of the saturated fat in human breast milk can be in the form of MCFAs. Sadly, many mothers produce very little.

If breast milk does not contain enough MCFAs, an infant can suffer from nutritional deficiency and become vulnerable to infectious illness. One of the major characteristics of human breast milk is its ability to protect infants from a myriad of infectious illnesses during a time when their immune systems are immature and incapable of adequately defending them. The antimicrobial substances in milk that protect the child from a world teaming with infectious germs and parasites are the MCFAs found in the triglycerides or fat molecules in the milk. There are some illnesses that even an adult with a healthy immune system may have difficulty fighting off. If the baby is not protected with an adequate amount of MCFAs in his or her milk, exposure to such an infection could result in serious illness.

It is important that mother's milk contain as much MCFAs as nature will allow. Given an ample supply of food containing MCFAs, a nursing mother will produce a milk rich in these health-promoting nutrients. While cow's milk and other dairy products contain small amounts, the foods richest in medium-chain fatty acids are the tropical oils, principally coconut oil.

The levels of these antimicrobial fatty acids can be as low as 3 to 4 percent, but when nursing mothers eat coconut products (shredded coconut, coconut milk, coconut oil, etc.) the levels of MCFAs in their milk increase significantly. For instance, eating 40 grams (about 3 tablespoons) of coconut oil in one meal can temporarily increase the lauric acid in the milk of a nursing mother from 3.9 percent to 9.6 percent after 14 hours. The content of caprylic and capric acids is also increased. If the mother consumes coconut oil every day while nursing, the MCFA content will be even greater.

Preparation by the mother should start before the baby is born. Pregnant women store fat to be used later in making their milk. After the baby is born, the fatty acids stored in the mother's body and supplied by her daily diet are used in the production of her milk. If she has eaten and continues to eat foods that supply ample amounts of MCFAs, particularly lauric acid and capric acid (the two most important antimicrobial medium-chain fatty acids), her milk will provide maximum benefit to her baby. These mothers can have as much as 18 percent of the saturated fatty acids in their milk in the form of lauric and capric acids. If, on the other hand, the mother did not eat foods containing MCFAs and does not eat them while nursing, her mammary glands will only be capable of producing about 3 percent lauric acid and 1 percent capric acid.

Vital nutrients and protectors found naturally in human milk, MCFAs are deadly enough to kill viruses yet gentle enough to nourish a premature infant to health. As we grow to adulthood and beyond, our bodies begin to wear down. As they do infants, MCFAs can help nourish and

protect us from infectious and degenerative disease. It appears that coconut oil provides many health benefits to those who are very young
and those who are very old and all those in between.

CROHN'S DISEASE

The inflammatory intestinal disease known as Crohn's is characterized
by diarrhea, abdominal pain, bleeding ulcers, bloody stools, anemia,
and weight loss. Ulcerations can occur anywhere along the digestive
tract from the mouth to the rectum. Ulcerative colitis is a similar disease
that affects the colon—the lower part of the intestinal tract. At times
these chronic conditions can become debilitating. The ability of the intestines to absorb food is hampered, which may lead to nutritional deficiencies. Sufferers find that certain foods aggravate symptoms, and
therefore they are constantly challenged to find foods that they can tolerate. Like many other chronic illnesses, Crohn's disease has no known
cure. Drugs can ease the symptoms, but if conditions become too severe, surgical removal of the infected organ is usually recommended.

However, interestingly enough, researchers have demonstrated the
benefits of coconut oil for patients with digestive problems, including
Crohn's disease, at least since the 1980s. The anti–inflammatory and healing effects of coconut oil apparently play a role in soothing and healing
the inflammation and injury in the digestive tract that are characteristic of Crohn's disease. Its antimicrobial properties also affect intestinal
health by killing troublesome microorganisms that may cause chronic
inflammation.

Dr. L. A. Cohen of the Naylor Dana Institute for Disease Prevention
in Valhalla, New York, notes the ease with which MCFAs in coconut
are digested and absorbed and says they "have found use in the clinic as
a means to provide high energy lipid to patients with disorders of lipid
digestion (pancreatitis), lipid absorption (Crohn's disease), and lipid trans-

port (chylomicron deficiency)." Eating coconut cookies has made an impact on Gerald Brinkley, a Crohn's disease sufferer for 30 years. "When I read that eating coconut macaroons could ease symptoms," Brinkley says, "I decided to try them myself. Coincidence or not, my symptoms have improved since I began eating two cookies a day."

Other anecdotal reports suggest that coconut may offer relief from symptoms and prevent digestive distress. Teresa Graedon, Ph.D., the co-author of *The People's Pharmacy Guide to Herbal and Home Remedies,* says that during the research for her book she heard enough testimonials about the benefit of using coconut for Crohn's disease that she was convinced that this is one home remedy that may have important medical significance and believes strongly that more research should be pursued in this area. I have also heard similar stories. For example, one case in Hawaii involved a small child who suffered from an intestinal problem so severe that almost any food, including milk, aggravated symptoms. The child was wasting away because he couldn't tolerate most of the foods he was given. A native Hawaiian told the mother to feed the child the "jelly" inside an immature coconut. She took the woman's advice, and the child thrived, eating a diet consisting primarily of coconut jelly (unripened coconut meat). Knowing what we know scientifically about the digestibility of coconut oil, it makes sense that it would be of benefit to those with digestive problems.

While the cause of Crohn's disease is still unknown, many doctors feel it is the result of a bacterial or viral infection. Stomach ulcers, for example, are caused primarily by the bacterium *H. pyloris.* It's possible that this bacterium or a similar one could also infect other areas of the digestive tract. Several studies have shown that the measles and mumps viruses might be involved in the development of Crohn's disease. In fact, a persistent low-grade measles infection in the intestine is common in many Crohn's and ulcerative colitis patients. Those who have had measles or mumps in the past and now suffer from some type of inflammatory bowel disease such as Crohn's disease or ulcerative colitis are likely to harbor a low-grade intestinal infection that the body has not been able to overcome. *H. pyloris* bacteria and the measles virus are both killed by the MCFAs in coconut oil. If the symptoms characteristic of Crohn's disease and ulcerative colitis are also caused by these or some other microorganism, then coconut oil may be beneficial in treating these conditions.

Eating macaroons to ease symptoms of Crohn's disease, as strange as it may sound, does have some scientific backing. For those who have Crohn's disease, ulcerative colitis, stomach ulcers, or other digestive problems, you don't have to eat coconut cookies to get relief—any food prepared with coconut oil or coconut milk would work just as well.

OSTEOPOROSIS

One of the advantages of using MCFAs in baby formula is that they help with the absorption of other nutrients. The absorption of calcium and magnesium, as well as amino acids, has been found to increase when infants are fed a diet containing coconut oil. Coconut oil has been used for the purpose of enhancing absorption and retaining calcium and magnesium in people when a deficiency of these minerals exists. This is one of the reasons why hospitals give premature and sick infants formulas containing MCFAs. It is also used to treat children suffering with rickets, which involves a demineralization and softening of the bones similar to osteoporosis in adults.

Regardless of your age, your bones can benefit from coconut oil. Dietary fats play a role in the formation of our bones. Researchers at Purdue University found that free radicals from oxidized vegetable oils interfere with bone formation, thus contributing to osteoporosis. They also discovered that antioxidants such as vitamin E protect the bones from free radicals. In addition, they found that saturated fats, like those in coconut oil, also act as antioxidants and protect the bones from destructive free radicals.

Fresh coconut, and perhaps virgin coconut oil, contains fatlike substances called sterols that are very similar in structure to pregnenolone.

Pregnenolone is a substance our bodies manufacture from sterols to make hormones such as dehydroepiandrosterone (DHEA) and progesterone. When women's bodies are in need of these hormones, pregnenolone is used as the starting material to make them. According to John Lee, M.D., the reason women are often plagued with osteoporosis as they get older is because they have an imbalance of progesterone to estrogen. Environmental estrogens from meat, milk, and pesticides dilute natural progesterone. In clinical practice Dr. Lee has had women use progesterone to increase their body's reserves of this hormone. Bone density tests before and after treatment showed a clear reversal of osteoporosis. Dr. Lee has outlined his findings in his book *What Your Doctor May Not Tell You About Menopause*. It is believed that pregnenolone, which is converted into progesterone in women, has the same bone-building effect. If this is true, the pregnenolonelike substances in coconut may also aid in maintaining hormone balance and promoting healthy bones.

This may be why populations that consume coconuts as a major part of their diets are rarely troubled by osteoporosis. For those who are concerned about developing osteoporosis as they get older, coconut oil may be useful in helping to slow down this degenerative process by improving mineral absorption, protecting the bones from free radicals, and maintaining hormone balance.

GALLBLADDER DISEASE

The purpose of the gallbladder is to store and regulate the use of bile. The function of bile in the digestive process is often given little notice, but it is essential. The liver produces bile at a relatively constant rate. As the bile is secreted, it drains into and is collected by the gallbladder. The gallbladder functions as a container to hold bile. Fats and oils in our foods stimulate the gallbladder to pump bile into the intestine. An adequate amount of bile is essential for the digestion of fats because it emulsifies or breaks the fat into small particles. Digestive enzymes from the pancreas can break the small particles of fat down into individual fatty acids, which can then be absorbed. Without bile, fat-digesting enzymes could not complete the job of digestion; this would lead to serious nutritional deficiencies and disease.

When the gallbladder is surgically removed, fat digestion is greatly hindered. Without the gallbladder, the bile, which is continually being secreted by the liver, slowly drains into the small intestine. The tiny amount of bile that drains directly from the liver into the intestine is not enough to function adequately in fat digestion when even moderate amounts of fat are consumed. This leads to malabsorption of fat-soluble vitamins and to digestive problems. Bile must be present in the intestine to properly absorb fat-soluble vitamins (vitamins A, D, E, and K and beta-carotene). The consequence of not getting enough of these vitamins may not be immediately noticeable but over time will manifest itself in a variety of ways.

Metabolism of MCFAs does not require bile or pancreatic enzymes, so someone who has had his or her gallbladder removed or who has trouble digesting fats would greatly benefit from the use of coconut oil.

VIRAL INFECTIONS

One of the most amazing benefits of coconut oil is its ability to kill disease-causing viruses. Antibiotics are useless against viruses, and antiviral drugs have only limited effectiveness. Medications used to treat viral infections are often accompanied by undesirable side effects. Coconut oil is a natural, harmless product that is gaining notice as a means to help prevent and even treat viral infections.

CHRONIC FATIGUE SYNDROME

Coconut oil may be one of the best solutions to chronic fatigue syndrome (CFS) currently available. Once considered an imaginary ailment, CFS is now recognized as a bona fide illness. While its cause is still pretty much a mystery, it has become a problem of growing concern. It is estimated that some 3 million Americans and 90 million people worldwide are affected by it.

This illness is characterized by a relatively sudden onset of extreme fatigue, often following an infectious illness. Symptoms may include any of the following: muscle weakness, headache, memory loss, mental confusion, recurring infections, low-grade fever, swollen lymph glands, severe exhaustion following moderate physical activity, depression, anxiety attacks, dizziness, rashes, allergies, and autoimmune reactions. Symptoms that persist for six months or more are a strong indication of CFS.

The degree and severity of symptoms often fluctuate. An afflicted person may temporarily "recover" and function normally for a while, only to relapse a short time later. Many people are affected without even realizing it. They assume their symptoms are due to age, stress, or seasonal illness, and they do nothing to solve the problem.

The exact cause of the illness is still unknown, and there is no standard medical test to detect it. Consequently, a cure has yet to be found. The current belief is that CFS does not have a single cause but is the result of many factors. Some believe it is the result of multiple chronic infections that depress the immune system and drain the body of energy. Poor nutrition, excessive stress, food and environmental toxins, and chronic infections all combine to lower immune function and drain energy. Many people believe that a depressed immune system is the primary cause of the problem.

Any number of viruses, bacteria, fungi, or parasites can contribute to chronic fatigue. The most likely causes are the herpes virus, the Epstein-Barr virus, candida, and giardia. Some infections, especially viruses such as herpes, can persist for a lifetime. For example, herpes can cause fever blisters and genital lesions. The blisters may disappear temporarily, only to reappear occasionally when the efficiency of the body's immune system drops, especially as a result of stress.

The Epstein-Barr virus is a member of the herpes family that causes mononucleosis; it is often called the kissing disease because it can be transmitted this way. Once inside the body it attacks the white blood cells. Recovery takes four to six weeks with rest. The body needs this length of time to allow the immune system to overcome the virus. For two to three months afterward, patients often feel depressed, lack energy, and feel sleepy throughout the day. This condition may persist at a chronic level, giving rise to CFS.

Cold and flu viruses can cause chronic infections that may contribute to chronic fatigue. Often people with viral infections are given antibiotics. There is no antibiotic that can kill a virus. When we come down with a cold, flu, or other viral infection, the only thing we can do is take it easy and let our immune system handle the job. Doctors often give people who are suffering from viral infections antibiotics because there is nothing else they can do. The antibiotics have no more effect than a placebo—to make the patient feel he or she is doing something to hasten recovery. This has been the standard practice among doctors for years. The problem with this, besides wasting patients' money and subjecting them to worthless medications, is that the antibiotics may do some harm. One of the side effects of antibiotic use is the development of candidiasis. Antibiotics kill friendly bacteria in the intestinal tract that compete for space with yeast, thus keeping candida numbers low and relatively harmless. If these bacteria are killed by antibiotic use, yeasts are able to multiply unrestrained, causing a systemic candida infection. Candida can become chronic, burdening the immune system, draining the body's energy, and leading to prolonged feelings of fatigue and ill health.

As mentioned in chapter 4, giardia infections produce symptoms often diagnosed as chronic fatigue syndrome. Low-grade bacterial infections may also drain the body's energy, causing chronic fatigue. Low-grade infections can be nearly impossible to diagnose accurately. If a virus is part of the cause, little can be done, as there are no drugs that can cure viral illnesses. Giving the wrong type of medication can make matters worse, so experimenting with antibiotics and other drugs is not a good solution.

What's the answer? Coconut oil may provide a vital solution to chronic fatigue syndrome. The fatty acids in coconut oil can kill herpes,

Epstein-Barr viruses, candida, giardia, and a variety of other infectious organisms, any of which could contribute to chronic fatigue. Some doctors believe it is not the particular germ or organism that matters; any combination of factors or conditions that depress the immune system can lead to CFS. According to them, the key to overcoming CFS is strengthening the immune system. Again, coconut oil may be the solution. Coconut oil supports the immune system by ridding the body of

---

"I never thought I was troubled with chronic fatigue syndrome. I was healthy. I ate what I considered a good diet—low in fat, lots of fruits, vegetables, and whole grains. But I noticed as I was approaching my mid-forties my level of energy was decreasing rapidly. Even modest amounts of yard work became a drudgery. After a couple of hours I came in exhausted, and it took me two days to recover. By 8 p.m. every day I was exhausted, even though I have a desk job. I found myself going to bed earlier and earlier. Life was slowing down, and I missed the energy I once had. I assumed that what I was experiencing was just the consequence of growing older and left it at that.

"But then I began to wonder. I saw other people, much older than me, who were more physically active and had much more energy. I then suspected something was wrong. I began to seek ways to improve my health. I learned about coconut and began to eat it in place of other oils. I did this not to cure any illness but simply to improve my overall health. It was several months later when I noticed that the energy I used to have began to return. I no longer wanted to go to sleep at 8 p.m. but stayed up till 11 without a problem. I got less sleep but had more energy. Improvement came so gradually that I didn't notice the change until after several months. And it wasn't until later that I even thought it might be related to coconut oil. Since I've been using coconut oil I have not been lethargic during the day, as I was in the past; I have more energy and accomplish more. I feel really good."

—*Brian M.*

harmful microorganisms, thus relieving stress on the body. With fewer harmful organisms taxing the body's energy, the immune system can function better.

Coconut oil also provides a quick source of energy and stimulates metabolism. This boost in energy not only lifts the spirit but promotes faster healing. The higher the body's metabolism, the more efficient the immune system and the more quickly the body can heal and repair itself. It's like a carpenter doing some repairs on your house. If he is tired and slow, it will take a long time to do the job, but if he is energetic and anxious to complete the task, it will take a fraction of the time. When metabolism is functioning at a higher level, our cells are like an energized carpenter anxious to complete the repairs, while depressed metabolism causes the cells to work more slowly, and consequently healing and repair proceed more slowly.

AIDS PREVENTION AND TREATMENT

After more than two decades of research, the AIDS epidemic is still going strong. Drugs have been developed to help slow down the progress of the disease, but, as is the case with other viruses, there is no cure. But there is hope. One of the most exciting and active areas of research with MCFAs is in the treatment of those infected with HIV, which, like many other microorganisms, has a lipid membrane that is vulnerable to MCFAs.

In the 1980s researchers discovered that the medium-chain fatty acids, specifically lauric and capric acids, were effective in killing HIV in lab cultures. This opened the door to a possible treatment for HIV/ AIDS that was far safer than the antiviral drugs currently being used.

One of the problems with the antiviral drugs used to fight HIV is that they have undesirable side effects, including muscle wasting, nausea, vomiting, anorexia, bone marrow suppression, ulcerations, hemorrhaging, skin rash, anemia, fatigue, and altered mental function. Another problem is that the AIDS virus can grow resistant to the drugs, often becoming invulnerable to them. The specific combination of viral resistance varies from patient to patient. To fight these resistant strains of superviruses, doctors use a hit–or–miss approach by brewing potent AIDS drug cock-tails. The more drugs used, the greater the risk of undesirable side effects.

Unlike the standard drugs used to treat HIV, which attack the virus's genetic material, medium–chain fatty acids simply break the virus apart. Much like the other fatty acids that make up the virus's lipid membrane, the MCFAs are absorbed by the virus; this weakens the membrane un-til it breaks apart, killing the virus. It is unlikely that the virus can de-velop an immunity to this mechanism, so MCFAs can attack and kill any of the strains of HIV, even the genetically drug–resistant superviruses.

Over the years many HIV-infected individuals have reported a de-crease in their viral load (the number of viruses in the blood) and an im-provement in overall health after eating coconut or drinking coconut milk. Some have reported lowering their viral loads to nondetectable levels after eating coconut for only a few weeks.

The first clinical study on the effectiveness of coconut oil to treat HIV patients was reported by Cornrado Dayrit, M.D., emeritus pro-fessor of pharmacology at the University of the Philippines and for-mer president of the National Academy of Science and Technology in the Philippines. In this study, 14 HIV patients, ages 22 to 38, were separated into three groups. None of the patients received any other anti-HIV treatment during the study. The treatment they were testing compared monolaurin (the monoglyceride of lauric acid found in co-conut oil) and pure coconut oil. One group (four patients) was given 22 grams of monolaurin a day. The second group (five patients) was given 7.2 grams of monolaurin. The third group (five patients) was given 3½ tablespoons of coconut oil. The coconut oil given to the third group contained about the same quantity of lauric acid as was supplied by the monolaurin in the first group. After three months of treatment, the vi-ral load had decreased in seven of the patients. After six months, when the study was completed, 9 out of the 14 patients had a decreased viral count (two in the first group, four in the second, and three in the third). Eleven of the patients had regained weight and appeared to be improving. This study confirmed the anecdotal reports that coconut oil has anti-HIV effects and has provided solid clinical evidence that both monolaurin and coconut oil are effective in fighting HIV. Additional research is currently underway to further study the use of monolaurin and coconut oil to treat HIV/AIDS.

Unfortunately, the ready availability and low cost of coconut oil and its derivative fatty acids are reasons why research into its use as a treatment for AIDS and other viral illnesses has been slow. There is little monetary incentive for pharmaceutical companies to fund research on a natural, readily available substance that they cannot protect with a patent and charge exorbitant prices for. Currently the cost of standard medications for one person to control HIV can reach over $15,000 a year. If all the hundreds of thousands of people who are infected by this virus spend anywhere near this amount, you can easily see the enormous amount of money the pharmaceutical companies pull in. It is no wonder they are reluctant to support a treatment that threatens to end this flood of cash.

Individuals with HIV often suffer from nutritional deficiencies and recurrent infections. Resistance to infectious illness decreases as the disease progresses. Opportunistic microorganisms such as cytomegalovirus, candida, cryptosporidium, and others quickly take root. In time, the body is devastated so greatly by infection that survival is impossible. The fatty acids in coconut oil not only offer the possibility of reducing the HIV load but kill other harmful organisms as well. Combined with the fact that lauric acid and other MCFAs improve digestion and energy production, the result is better overall health.

Current research suggests that individuals infected with HIV progress more rapidly to AIDS when they have a higher viral load. Reducing the viral load to undetectable levels greatly increases the patient's chances of avoiding the disease and reduces the chance of infecting others. A recent study by researchers from Johns Hopkins University showed that the number of individual viruses in the person determines the degree to which the virus can be passed on to others. The study found that someone with 200,000 virus copies (individual viruses per mm of blood) is 2.5 times more likely to spread HIV than someone with only 2,000 copies. The researchers found no transmission of the virus at all by infected people who carried less than 1,500 copies of the virus.

In September 1996 AIDS patient Chris Dafoe of Cloverdale, Indiana, figured his time was running out. He'd lost a great deal of weight, lacked energy, and felt worse and worse with each passing day. The thing that drove the nail into his coffin was the lab results. The report showed he had a viral load of over 600,000—an indication of rampant HIV infection and a sign that he didn't have too much time left to live. So he made arrangements for his funeral, paying all expenses up front. Before he died, however, and while he still had some strength left, he wanted to take one last vacation—a dream vacation to the jungles of South America. He flew to the tiny Republic of Surinam and wound his way into the jungle, where he stayed briefly among a group of Indians. While there, he ate the same foods as the natives. Every day he was served a dish of cooked coconut prepared by the natives.

"The Indian Chief told me," says Dafoe, "that they use the coconut as the basis for all their medicines. They also use the milk from the inside of the coconut and also use other plants and herbs from the jungle to make medicines. They eat cooked coconut every morning to help prevent illness." While there, Dafoe's health took a turn for the better, his strength and energy increased, and he regained 32 pounds. Home again, six weeks later he went in for another lab test. This time the results showed his viral load had plummeted to undetectable levels. The HIV virus that had once flooded his body was no longer measurable.

He continues eating cooked coconut for breakfast every day, mixing it with hot cereal. He is convinced that it keeps the virus under control and allows him to enjoy good health. With a zest for life he says, "I feel great. I have more energy than ever."

Currently some researchers recommended that HIV-infected individuals consume the equivalent of 24–28 grams of lauric acid a day in order to significantly reduce their viral load. This would amount to about 3½ tablespoons (50 grams) of coconut oil. While it is not yet known if lauric acid may one day be a cure for AIDS, it has been proven to reduce the HIV load in those individuals who are infected by the virus, allowing them to live more normal lives and greatly reducing the risk of their transmitting the virus to others. It may be equally able to protect and possibly prevent infection in the first place if a person has sufficient lauric acid in his or her daily diet and low exposure to HIV.

OTHER SERIOUS ILLNESSES

When I first started digging through the medical literature searching for information about coconut oil I was amazed at the multitude of studies that showed benefits from its use. Studies showed that coconut oil could be of benefit for those concerned about cancer, diabetes, liver disease, kidney disease, prostate enlargement, and even epilepsy.

CANCER

If you are a woman, your chance of developing breast cancer is one in eight. If you are a man, your chance of getting prostate cancer is one in nine. One out of every three people alive today in the United States will eventually get some form of cancer during his or her lifetime. Cancer is second only to heart disease as the leading cause of death. Like heart disease, there is no sure cure. Often the treatment is as bad as the disease. The best defense is prevention, and most forms of cancer are preventable.

Every single one of us has cancerous cells in our bodies. The reason we don't all develop cancer and die is because the immune system destroys these renegade cells before they can get out of hand. As long as the immune system is functioning the way it was designed to, we need not worry about cancer. There are several things you can do to improve the efficiency of your immune system and help prevent cancer, such as eating a healthy diet, getting regular exercise, reducing stress, getting proper rest, and such. You should also avoid those things that promote cancer, such as smoking and consuming heat-damaged vegetable oils. As noted in chapter 2, processed vegetable oils depress the immune system and create free radicals that can promote cancer. Another thing you can do to strengthen your immune system is to eat coconut oil on a regular basis. Consuming coconut oil, especially in place of most other oils, can greatly reduce your chances of developing cancer.

We are continually surrounded by troublesome germs, many of which find entrance into our bodies. The white blood cells of our immune system constantly battle invading microbes as well as clean out diseased and cancerous cells. When exposure to germs is excessive or when the immune system is under stress, the white blood cells become overworked. When the immune system is under stress, it is unable to effectively clean out cancerous cells. When this happens, cancerous cells can grow and spread without restraint.

The antimicrobial properties of the MCFAs in coconut oil aid the body in eliminating disease-causing germs, thus relieving stress on the immune system. The MCFAs take over the job of killing many of the invading microbes. With fewer germs around to cause trouble, white blood cells are free to seek out and destroy cancerous cells. In this manner, coconut oil aids the body in defending itself against germs by allowing the white blood cells to focus their attention on cleaning out toxins and cancerous cells. So a major benefit of coconut oil in the fight against cancer is to reduce stress on the immune system, which in turn allows the white blood cells to function more efficiently so that cancerous cells don't have a chance to run amok.

Coconut oil not only assists the white blood cells but may also take an active part in fighting some forms of cancer. Dr. Robert L. Wickremasinghe, head of the serology division at the Medical Research Institute in Sri Lanka, reports that coconut oil appears to possess anti-carcinogenic properties. Researchers have shown that coconut oil inhibits the induction of carcinogenic agents that cause colon as well as mammary (breast) tumors in test animals (Reddy, 1992, and Cohen and Thompson, 1987). Many vegetable oils promote cancer because they are easily oxidized to form carcinogenic free radicals (Hopkins, 1981). MCFAs have an antioxidantlike effect that prevents free-radical reactions and appears to provide protection, at least in the case of breast and colon cancer.

DIABETES

One of the many plagues of modern society is diabetes. The incidence of diabetes has risen over the last century to make it the sixth biggest killer in America. Diabetes not only can cause death but also can lead to kidney disease, heart disease, high blood pressure, stroke, cataracts, nerve damage, hearing loss, and blindness. It is estimated that 45 percent of the population is at risk of developing diabetes.

Diabetes is all about sugar in our bodies, otherwise known as blood glucose. Every cell in our bodies must have a constant source of glucose in order to fuel metabolism. Our cells use glucose to power processes such as growth and repair. When we eat a meal, the digestive system converts much of our food into glucose, which is released into the bloodstream. The hormone insulin, which is secreted by the pancreas gland, moves glucose from the blood and funnels it into the cells so it can be used as fuel. If the cells are unable to get adequate amounts of glucose, as is the case in diabetes, they can literally starve to death and cause tissues and organs to degenerate.

There are two major forms of diabetes: Type I and Type II. Type I, also referred to as insulin-dependent or juvenile diabetes, usually begins in childhood and results from the inability of the pancreas to make adequate amounts of insulin. Type II diabetes is known as non-insulin-dependent or adult-onset diabetes because it usually appears in older adults. In Type II diabetes the pancreas may secrete a normal amount of insulin, but the cells are unable to absorb it. Insulin acts like a key to a lock. It goes to the cells and unlocks the door to allow glucose to enter. If the lock is made of cheap materials and breaks, the key no longer works, and the door remains locked. This is essentially what happens with Type II diabetes. In both types of diabetes the level of glucose in the blood is elevated, while cells are deprived.

In Type I the pancreas is incapable of producing enough insulin to adequately shuttle glucose to all the cells in the body. Treatment involves insulin injections one or more times a day, along with adherence to a strict low-sugar diet. About 90 percent of diabetics are of Type II, and 85 percent of them are overweight. Diet plays a key role in both the onset of the disease and its control. The types of foods we eat can either promote or protect us from diabetes.

In the Pacific Islands, diabetes is unheard-of among those people who eat traditional diets. But when they abandon their native foods and adopt Western ways, the incidence of diabetes rises. An interesting example of this has occurred on the island of Nauru in the South Pacific. Subsisting for centuries on a diet composed primarily of bananas, yams, and coconuts, the people lived totally free from diabetes. Phosphate deposits discovered on the island brought an influx of wealth and a change in lifestyle. The islanders replaced the coconut and yams they had eaten for centuries with foods made from refined flour, sugar, and processed vegetable oils. The result was the emergence of a never-before-seen disease—diabetes. According to the World Health Organization, up to half of the urbanized Nauru population age 30-64 are now diabetic.

Doctors have been able to help patients control diabetes by putting them on a low-fat, high-carbohydrate diet. The diet restricts total fat intake to 30 percent or less of calories. Complex carbohydrates such as whole grains and vegetables make up 50 to 60 percent of calories. Simple carbohydrates such as refined flour and sugar are to be avoided. The reason for this is because simple carbohydrates can put undue strain on the pancreas and quickly raise blood sugar to dangerous levels. The reason for reducing fat as well as sweets is to promote weight loss. Since excess weight is of primary concern with diabetes, losing it is a priority. Another reason for the low-fat diet is to reduce the risk of heart disease, which is a common consequence of diabetes. Probably the best reason for keeping fat to a minimum is that some fats, particularly oxidized fats, not only promote diabetes but may actually cause it.

Researchers have discovered that the overconsumption of refined vegetable oils leads to diabetes. As far back as the 1920s, Dr. S. Sweeney produced reversible diabetes in all of his medical school students by feeding them a high-vegetable-oil diet for 48 hours. None of the students had previously been diabetic. More recently, researchers have been able to cause test animals to develop diabetes by feeding them diets high in polyunsaturated fat (Parekh, 1998). Simply restricting fat intake in diabetic animals has shown to reverse Type II diabetes. Likewise, clinical studies with humans on low-fat diets also show reversal of the disease. Many studies have shown low-fat diets to be effective in controlling diabetes.

The current recommendation is to limit all fats. Monounsaturated fats, such as olive oil, don't seem to adversely affect diabetes and so are allowed in moderation, but because all fats, including olive oil, are high in calories, they are discouraged. Saturated fat is restricted because it is believed to increase risk of heart disease. The biggest culprit, however, seems to be polyunsaturated oil. Studies have shown that when polyunsaturated fats from the diet are incorporated into cellular structure, the cell's ability to bind with insulin decreases, thus lowering its ability to get glucose. In other words, the "locks" on the cells that open the door for glucose to enter degrade when too much polyunsaturated oil is consumed in the diet. Insulin is then unable to open the door. Polyunsaturated oils are easily oxidized and damaged by free radicals. Fats of all types, including polyunsaturated oils, are used as building blocks for cell membranes. Oxidized polyunsaturated fats in the cell membrane can adversely affect the cell's function, including its ability to allow hormones, glucose, and other substances to flow in and out of the cell. Therefore, a diet high in refined polyunsaturated vegetable oils promotes diabetes. A diet low in such oils helps to alleviate symptoms. Because all fats also promote weight gain, it's best to avoid them as much as possible.

There is one fat that diabetics can eat without fear. That fat is coconut oil. Not only does it not contribute to diabetes but it helps regulate blood sugar, thus lessening the effects of the disease. MCFA can supply needed energy to cells without adversely affecting blood sugar or insulin levels. Because coconut oil can also help regulate metabolism (see chapter 5), it can help the body burn more calories, causing weight loss and helping to regulate diabetes.

As mentioned earlier in this chapter, coconut oil puts less of a demand on the enzyme production of the pancreas. This lessens the stress on the pancreas during mealtime when insulin is produced most heavily, thus allowing the organ to function more efficiently. Coconut oil also helps supply energy to cells because it is easily absorbed without the need of enzymes or insulin. It has been shown to improve insulin secretion and utilization of blood glucose. Coconut oil in the diet enhances insulin action and improves binding affinity compared to other oils. The *Journal of the Indian Medical Association* has reported that Type II diabetes in India has increased as the people have abandoned traditional oils, like coconut oil, in favor of polyunsaturated vegetable oils, which have been promoted as "heart-friendly." The authors comment on the link between polyunsaturated oils and diabetes and recommend increasing coconut oil consumption as a means to prevent diabetes.

LIVER DISEASE

The liver is one of the most important organs in the body. It detoxifies, builds proteins and fats, secretes hormones, stores vitamins and minerals, produces bile necessary for digestion, and performs a hundred or so other functions vital to maintaining proper health. When the liver becomes diseased, any number of health-threatening conditions can arise. Two of the most common liver problems we hear about are hepatitis and cirrhosis. Both can be fatal. A number of different conditions can produce hepatitis; among them are alcohol, drugs, viruses, and bacteria.

Three types of hepatitis, designated as hepatitis A, B, and C, are caused by viral infections. Two of the liver's most destructive enemies are viruses and free radicals—both of which can be protected against by the regular consumption of coconut oil.

Hepatitis A virus is found in feces and is transmitted by poor sanitation and hygiene. It is estimated that in the United States, about 40 percent of young adults have been exposed to the hepatitis A virus. In some parts of the world where hygiene is poor, almost everyone has been exposed. Hepatitis B and C viruses are most often passed by sexual contact or needle-sharing among drug abusers. They are both less common than hepatitis A. In parts of Africa and Asia up to 20 percent of the population is infected by hepatitis B. In the United States the rate is about 1 percent. Hepatitis C is the most severe of the three and often leads to liver cirrhosis.

Chronic hepatitis, alcohol or drug abuse, or infection may lead to cirrhosis. Liver cirrhosis is a degenerative condition characterized by massive tissue destruction and scarring. The liver damage that alcoholics and hepatitis patients experience is caused largely by the destructive action of free radicals. The destruction caused by free radicals seriously affects the liver's ability to function and if left untreated can lead to organ failure and death.

Researchers have been finding coconut oil to be of great benefit to liver health. The MCFAs are immediately funneled from the digestive tract to the liver, where they can aid the organ in many ways. Viruses that cause hepatitis are deactivated by the MCFAs, thus aiding the immune system in fighting off dangerous infections.

MCFAs are resistant to free-radical formation and actually help prevent their formation in the liver. A study by H. Kono and others showed that MCFAs can prevent alcohol-induced liver injury by inhibiting free-radical formation. Several other studies have also shown that fatty acids, such as those found in coconut and palm kernel oils, protect the liver from alcohol-induced free-radical injury and tissue death, indicating that the use of these oils can not only prevent injury but even rejuvenate diseased tissue. Dr. A. Nanji and other researchers suggest using fatty acids (from tropical oils) as a dietary treatment for alcoholic liver disease.

PROSTATE ENLARGEMENT

If you are male, chances are you will suffer some type of prostate problem during your lifetime. The most common prostate problem is benign prostatic hyperplasia (BPH), or prostate enlargement. Nearly half of all men between the ages of 40 and 59, and as many as 90 percent of those in their seventies and eighties have some symptoms of BPH. It has become so bad that it's almost an invariable consequence of aging. Prostate enlargement, however, is not simply a result of aging; lifestyle and diet play an important role. This condition is only a major problem in westernized countries. Those men who live in less prosperous localities of the world where local foods are produced and consumed don't appear to be troubled by it as much. While the exact cause of BPH is unknown, recent lipid research has revealed that coconut oil may be beneficial in prevention and treatment.

It is believed that as men age, testosterone is converted into the male hormone dihydrotestosterone (DHT) and accumulates in the prostate gland. This hormone encourages the growth of prostate cells, which causes the prostate to enlarge and pinch off the urethra, the tube through which urine flows from the bladder. This causes frequent and impaired urination, especially at night, and is often associated with inflammation of the gland. While not normally cancerous, it sets the stage for such a condition to exist.

A logical treatment for BPH is to block the conversion of testosterone into DHT. The drug finasteride works on this principle and has been effective. Saw palmetto is a popular herbal remedy that also appears to block the toxic effect of excess DHT formation. The berries of this subtropical plant found in the southeastern part of the United States were used by native Indians of Florida and early settlers as a folk medicine to treat reproductive disorders, urinary diseases, and colds. In women it has been used to increase the supply of mother's milk and to relieve painful periods.

Studies show saw palmetto berries are very effective at reducing the effects of BPH and are remarkably safe. Compared with Proscar (a much-prescribed BPH drug), saw palmetto is more effective in reducing prostate symptoms. Numerous studies have shown saw palmetto extract to be effective in nearly 90 percent of patients, usually in a period of four to six weeks. In contrast, Proscar is effective in reducing the symptoms in less than 37 percent of patients after taking the drug for a full year. Saw palmetto has no adverse side effects. Proscar, on the other hand, may cause impotence, decreased libido, and birth defects. Saw palmetto has gained a reputation among both alternative and conventional health care professionals as an effective treatment for BPH. It is one herb that even conventional medicine recognizes as safe and effective.

Saw palmetto is a member of the palm family and a relative of the coconut, and its medicinal effects are derived primarily from fatty acids in the berries. Many of the fatty acids in saw palmetto berries are MCFAs similar to those in coconut. Dr. Jon Kabara, an expert in lipid (fat) bio-

> "I'm a nurse with a natural alternative wellness center in Missouri. I use virgin coconut oil as a foundational product for all of my clients. It is one of the most powerful supplements I have ever worked with (I have been in the healing arts for 30 years and natural approaches for 20 years) and I find it works great for all blood types and body types. My only caution is that it is very powerful and has the ability to detoxify your body quickly. A few of my clients have had to start out on a teaspoon and work up, due to the detoxification response being more intense than they wanted to experience. Most people I work with are able to use 3–4 tablespoons per day from the start, with amazing results in improved immune system, energy level, stabilized blood sugar, improved thyroid function, weight loss, more mental clarity, and improved emotional/mental stability. In addition to being a wonderful supplement, it is a basic food that should replace all other oils that one has been cooking with. I don't know of any other product that covers so many bases—and it tastes great too!"
>
> —*Marie D.*

chemistry, suggests that just as the fatty acids in saw palmetto berries inhibit the formation of DHT hormone, so should the fatty acids in coconut oil.

BETTER HEALTH WITH COCONUT OIL

Coconut has been used as both a food and a medicine for centuries in many cultures throughout the world. Traditional forms of medicine use coconut oil for a wide variety of health problems, ranging from the treatment of burns and constipation to gonorrhea and influenza. Modern medical research is now confirming the effectiveness of coconut oil for many of these conditions. Research over the past several decades has demonstrated that the medium-chain fatty acids in coconut oil are digested and metabolized differently from those of other fats. This difference gives the oil many health benefits obtained from no other source.

Medium-chain triglycerides in coconut oil don't require pancreatic enzymes or bile for digestion. They are easy to digest, making them ideal for infants, cystic fibrosis patients, and those who have digestive problems, including those with gallbladder disease and those who have had their gallbladders removed.

Coconut oil has been recommended for use in the treatment of malnutrition because it provides a quick and easy source of nutrition without taxing the enzyme systems of the body. It also improves the absorption of minerals (particularly calcium and magnesium) B vitamins, and fat-soluble vitamins (A,D, E, and K and beta-carotene), as well as some amino acids. The MCFAs in coconut oil are used by the body to produce energy, not make body fat. Coconut oil stimulates metabolism, increases energy, and improves thyroid function, all of which aid in reducing unwantd body fat. For these reasons, coconut oil has gained a reputation as being the world's only natural low-calorie fat. Researchers have recommended the oil as a means to prevent and even treat obesity.

Coconut oil is heart healthy. It does not negatively affect blood cholesterol, does not promote platelet stickiness that leads to blood clot formation, and does not collect in the arteries. Coconut oil possesses anti-inflammatory, antimicrobial, and antioxidant properties, all of which protect arteries from atherosclerosis and from heart disease. Those people around the world who consume the most coconut oil have the lowest rates of heart disease. This is true even for those populations who get as much as 50 percent of their daily calories from saturated fat, primarily from coconut oil.

The MCFAs possess powerful antimicrobial properties that kill a variety of disease-causing bacteria, fungi, viruses, and parasites, yet they do not harm friendly gut bacteria or contribute to antibiotic resistance. Coconut oil may be of great help to those with common infections such as influenza and candida as well as more serious problems like HIV.

Because of its resistance to free-radical formation and its ability to support the immune system, coconut oil may be useful in preventing or treating a wide assortment of conditions, many of which aren't even discussed in this book. Medical researchers and health care workers are discovering new health benefits associated with coconut oil all the time.

Currently, several clinics in the United States are testing the efficiency of a dietary supplement composed of monolaurin—a derivative of coconut oil. Doctors have reported remarkable results with patients. One female patient, for example, who suffered with ovarian cysts for 20 years began taking the supplement, and within one month the cysts began to shrink and disappear. In another case a man who had had hepatitis C for two decades was put on the supplement. After six months his viral load dropped from 1 million to nondetectable levels. He no longer needed supplemental oxygen to breathe. His liver enzymes became normal, and he was up and out of his wheelchair, living a normal life.

Researchers are also discovering that coconut oil may be useful in the treatment of kidney and bladder problems. For example, in a study where kidney failure was induced in test animals, those that were given coconut oil had fewer and less severe lesions and survived longer. The researchers concluded that coconut oil has a protective effect on the kidneys. Because of the antimicrobial effects of coconut oil, it may also be of benefit for any number of kidney and bladder infections. A woman came to see me complaining about a bladder infection that had first become noticeable that morning. I told her about coconut oil, and she began taking it orally immediately. Without any other treatment, the infection disappeared completely within two days. Since then I have recommended it to others with bladder infections with good results.

Another incredible use researchers have discovered for coconut oil is in the treatment of epilepsy. When added to the diet, MCFAs have proven to be effective in reducing epileptic seizures in children. D. L. Ross of the University of Minnesota Medical School showed that seizure

"During the past several months, I have been experiencing severe insomnia. I do not believe in taking drugs to assist in sleeping, but it had gotten so bad that I got a prescription from my doctor. On using the prescription (and I have only tried this a couple of times) I was still only able to increase my night's sleep from about two hours to about four, and after taking the sleeping pills I felt so much worse the next day that I had abandoned that as a solution to my problem. I have noticed that since using the coconut I am now getting a full eight hours' sleep. Also, the pain in my hands, vertebrae, and knees from arthritis have almost completely disappeared. I still have the occasional twinges in the knuckle in the little finger on my right hand, but I suspect that is because it has calcified.

"I almost feel foolish writing this, because I cannot quite believe that I have been the beneficiary of such incredible improvement from all my ails, just from consuming coconut milk and oil. I keep expecting the problems to return. Another benefit is that I have lost the chronic irritability that I have had for so long that I was beginning to think that I had a personality change. I can only attribute all of these things to the coconut oil, as nothing else about my life has changed."

—Rhea L.

frequency decreased by more than 50 percent in two-thirds of the children in his study during a 10-week treatment period. What an amazing health food!

As coconut oil becomes more widely used, we are certain to find many more health benefits with this wonder of nature. It's incredible that some people still ignorantly criticize coconut oil as being unhealthy. Hopefully, the information in this book will help educate doctors, dieticians, and the general public about the healing miracles of coconut oil.

8

EAT YOUR WAY TO BETTER HEALTH

The regular use of coconut oil can make a dramatic difference in your life. If you are overweight it can help you lose excess body fat; if you have digestive problems it will help with that as well. Coconut oil can help you feel and look younger, give you more energy, protect you from infections and illnesses, and help prevent many degenerative conditions such as heart disease and cancer. Coconut oil is truly one of nature's most remarkable health tonics.

You can begin enjoying the benefits of coconut without making any drastic changes in your normal way of living. In fact, incorporating coconut into your life can be done with just three simple steps: (1) use coconut oil in your cooking and get rid of all other vegetable oils in your diet, (2) eat coconut and coconut products as a regular part of your diet, and (3) apply coconut oil directly to your skin and hair in order to absorb its healing benefits directly into your body. This chapter will help you learn how to incorporate coconut oil and products into your lifestyle. In the next chapter, I have provided many delicious recipes that include coconut and coconut oil, as well as instructions on how to use coconut oil as part of your beauty regimen. But first you need to understand what the good sources of coconut oil are and exactly how

Essential Fatty Acids

To be healthy and avoid deficiency disease, you must get all the nutrients your body needs. Fats are important nutrients and essential fatty acids (EFAs) are necessary for good health. Some of the fatty acids are classified as being "essential" because our bodies cannot make them from other nutrients—we must get them from our foods. The two basic essential fats are omega-6 (linoleic) and omega-3 (alpha-linolenic) fatty acids. Medium-chain fatty acids, like those found in coconut oil, are also important and are considered *conditionally essential:* that is, under certain circumstances they are just as important as other essential fatty acids.

The EFAs are contained in most vegetable oils but are often damaged by refining and processing or destroyed by free radicals. Therefore, conventionally processed vegetable oils are inferior sources of EFAs. In addition, trans fatty acids from hydrogenated oils, including margarine and shortening, block or interfere with the body's utilization of EFAs. For these reasons, if you eat conventionally processed vegetable oils and hydrogenated oils you may be deficient in EFA.

You can get the EFAs your body needs directly from your foods, unrefined cold-pressed vegetable oils, or dietary supplements. Coconut oil, however, has a very small percentage of these fats (only 2 percent). A benefit of using coconut oil in your daily diet is that MCFAs work synergistically with the essential fatty acids, improving the body's utilization of these fats. A diet rich in coconut oil can enhance the efficiency of essential fatty acids by as by as much as 100 percent (Gerster, 1998). Not only that, but coconut oil also acts as an antioxidant, protecting EFAs from destructive oxidation inside the body.

The World Health Organization says we need to get about 3 percent of our daily calories from the essential fatty acids. There is no set minimum for the MCFAs, although we know infants probably need somewhere around 5–10 percent of calories from this source. We also know from island populations that people can get as much as 50 percent of their calories from coconut oil without harm and that this probably provides them with much benefit. So it appears that for optimal health we should consume a small amount of EFAs along with a significantly larger amount of MCFAs.

much coconut oil you will need in order to take advantage of all of its healing benefits.

SOURCES OF TROPICAL OILS

In order to gain the marvelous benefits available from MCFAs, we must eat those foods that contain them. The only significant dietary sources of MCFAs are whole milk, butter, and particularily palm kernel and coconut. The butterfat in cow's milk contains a small amount of MCFAs, but most milk and dairy products nowadays are low-fat or nonfat and therefore provide essentially none of these health-giving fatty acids. Butter only consists of about 6 percent MCFAs. The better sources of MCFAs are the tropical oils. Palm kernel oil contains 58 percent MCFAs, but the only place you will find this oil is as an ingredient in a few commercially prepared foods. Coconut oil contains 63 percent MCFAs, and fresh or dried coconut meat has 33 percent fat. Coconut milk is 17 to 24 percent fat. So coconut products—the meat, oil, and milk—are by far the most readily available and richest dietary sources of MCFAs.

THE TROPICAL OILS

Palm, palm kernel, and coconut oils are referred to as the tropical oils. They come from different species of palm trees. The tropical oils have similar characteristics when used in food preparation. Their nutritional and fatty acid content, however, are somewhat different. All the tropical oils are rich in valuable nutrients and health-promoting fatty acids. Unlike most other vegetable oils, the tropical oils are composed primarily of saturated fatty acids. The unique thing about the tropical oils, especially palm kernel and coconut oils, is that their saturated fatty acids are predominantly of the health-promoting medium-chain variety.

Palm and palm kernel oil are two different oils that come from the same species of tree, one from the seed and the other from the husk surrounding the seed. Palm oil is obtained from the husk by steaming, heating, or pressing. Unlike other tropical oils, palm oil has only a small amount of MCFAs. Palm kernel oil is extracted from the seed. The seed kernel is only an inch or so in diameter and somewhat resembles a miniature coconut. The appearance of the two oils is quite different. Palm oil has a deep orange-red color that is due to the high concentration of beta-carotene and other carotenoids. Palm kernel oil, like coconut oil, is derived from the white meat inside the shell of the seed and is pure white in appearance.

Palm and palm kernel oils are not readily available to the average consumer in most Western countries; they're most commonly used by the food processing industry. You may run across some palm oil, however. A few ethnic or specialty stores carry it for household use. Some companies are now selling it as a nonhydrogenated shortening. Coconut oil, however, is commonly sold for kitchen use and is rapidly increasing in popularity because it is the richest natural source of health-promoting MCFAs. Coconut oil is available in most health food stores and is sold by many mail order companies.

RBD AND VIRGIN COCONUT OIL

Coconut oil is produced from the seed of a species of palm tree different from the one that produces palm and palm kernel oils. Because of the high oil content (33 percent), extracting oil from coconuts is a relatively simple process and has been the major source of vegetable oil for people in the tropics for thousands of years. Traditionally the oil is extracted from either fresh or dried coconut by boiling and/or fermentation. When boiled in water, the oil separates from the meat and floats to the surface, where it can easily be scooped out. Fermentation allows the

oil and water to separate out naturally. The juice, or "milk," of the coconut is squeezed out of the meat. The milk is then allowed to ferment
for 24–36 hours. During this time, the oil separates from the water. The
oil is removed and then heated slightly for a short time to evaporate all
moisture. Heat such as this isn't harmful because the oil is very stable
even under moderately high temperatures.

There are many different methods of processing coconut oil that affect the quality, appearance, flavor, and aroma of the finished product.
Coconut oil is commonly divided into two broad categories—"refined,
bleached, and deodorized" (RBD) and "virgin." The difference between the two is in the amount of processing the oil undergoes. The
term "virgin" is not an official classification; it simply signifies an oil
that has been subjected to less intense refining—lower temperatures and
no chemicals.

The RBD oil is typically made from dried coconut, known as copra,
which is made by drying coconut in the sun, smoking it, heating it in a
kiln, or some combination of these. Oil made from copra is the most
common coconut oil used in the cosmetic and food industries. While
high temperatures and chemical solvents are used to produce this oil, it
is still considered a healthy dietary oil because the fatty acids in coconut
oil are not harmed in the refining process. The RBD oil is generally
colorless, tasteless, and odorless. Many people prefer this type of oil for
all-purpose cooking and body-care needs because it doesn't affect the
flavor of foods or leave an odor when used on the skin.

Most virgin coconut oils are made from fresh coconuts, not copra.
The oil is extracted by any number of methods: boiling, fermentation,
refrigeration, mechanical press, or centrifuge. Since high temperatures
and chemical solvents are not used, the oil retains its naturally occurring
phytochemicals (plant chemicals), which produce a distinctive coconut
taste and smell.

Virgin coconut oil made from fresh coconuts is a pure white when
the oil is solidified, or crystal clear like water when liquefied. The RBD
oil made from copra can be just as clear and white. You often can't tell

the difference between them just by looking. The way to distinguish between them is by the smell and taste. The RBD oils are bland. Virgin oils have a delightfully mild coconut flavor and aroma.

There are some oils that may be labeled "virgin" and are made from sun-dried copra rather than fresh coconut. These are called cochin oils. They have undergone less processing than most RBD oils. This doesn't mean they are more natural than refined copra oil (RBD); they are actually a lesser or inferior quality. The term "cochin" is derived from a place in India, Cochin, where cheap copra oil is popular. These oils have a strong smell and taste and are slightly discolored. When coconut is dried in the open air it is common for the copra to become moldy. The oil made from this type of copra has a yellowish or gray color because of the mold. The mold residue is considered harmless because the heat used in the processing has rendered it sterile. You can tell the difference between these oils and true virgin coconut oil by the color. Because cochin oil contains a higher level of impurities than other coconut oils it has a relatively short shelf life, about six months. Cochin oil is used mostly in the making of soaps and cosmetics. It is often sold as a cooking oil in Asian markets.

Coconut oil is sold in various-sized bottles. Fourteen- to 16-ounce bottles are typical. I buy mine by the gallon. Often people ask me what type or brand of oil they should use. I have a simple answer. Buy the one that tastes best to you. If you don't like the taste of a certain brand, try another. There is a wide difference in the taste of oils. If you are going to use the oil frequently, you want one that you will be happy with. Some people don't like the taste of coconut in all their foods. For these people I recommend they try one of the tasteless brands. Personally I like the taste of coconut and love the delicate taste and aroma of virgin coconut oil. It costs a little more than the other types, but it is worth it. Some brands of oil have a strong flavor. I don't care for them, but some people like them.

At present, good-quality coconut oil is still difficult to find in some areas. The best places to look for it are in health food stores. If your local store doesn't carry it, ask them to order it for you. If you can't find a source of coconut oil in your area, check the resources listed at the back of this book.

HOW MUCH COCONUT OIL DO YOU NEED?

Researchers have yet to determine precisely how much coconut oil is needed daily to gain the optimal health benefit. However, on the basis of the amount of MCFAs found in human breast milk, which is known to be effective in its role of protecting and nourishing infants, we can estimate the amount that may be suitable for adults. On the basis of this premise, an adult of average size would need 3½ tablespoons (50 grams) of coconut oil a day to equal the proportion of MCFAs a nursing baby receives. The same amount of MCFAs can be obtained from 10 ounces of coconut milk or 7 ounces of raw coconut (about half a whole coconut).

Studies have shown that the antimicrobial effects of MCFAs increases with the quantity used, so the greater the number of these infection-fighting fatty acids available in our bodies, the greater our protection.

Daily Dose Comparison

The amount of medium-chain fatty acids that is believed to be necessary for optimal health can be obtained from a variety of coconut products. The following all contain about the same amount of MCFA.

3½ tablespoons pure coconut oil
7 ounces fresh coconut meat (about half a coconut)
2¾ cups dried, shredded coconut
10 ounces coconut milk

Eating more should provide greater health benefits, not only in preventing illness but in improving digestion and nutrient absorption, protecting against heart disease, and so on.

It is not known for certain whether it is possible to consume too much coconut. Coconut oil is essentially nontoxic to humans. It is considered safer than soy, which many people eat by the pound. The FDA has included coconut oil on its list of foods that are "generally regarded as safe." This is an exclusive list. Only those foods that have passed stringent testing and have a history of safe usage can qualify for inclusion on the GRAS list. We know that certain island populations consume large amounts of coconut oil, as much as 10 tablespoons a day, and have excellent health. This is far more than you would normally want to eat, so you probably don't need to worry about eating too much. Several clinical studies have shown MCFA levels up to at least 1 gram per each kilogram of body weight to be safe. For a 150-pound person that would equate to 5 tablespoons. For a 200-pound person that would be 6.5 tablespoons.

My recommendation is for an adult to consume 2–4 tablespoons of coconut oil daily. This dose could be achieved through cooking, taking it as a supplement, or by applying it directly to the skin. Incorporating coconut oil into your cooking is the most palatable way to get the daily dose, and it is the easiest way to measure how much you are actually using, so it is the first step in my coconut lifestyle plan. But I do provide guidelines here for taking the oil as a supplement. Step 3 of my plan involves coconut oil applications to the skin.

COOKING WITH COCONUT OIL

Replacing the cooking oils you currently use with coconut oil is the easy first step to adding MCFAs to your diet without increasing your total fat intake. Eliminate all margarine, shortening, and processed vegetable oils from your diet. Olive oil and butter are okay, but use coconut oil whenever possible. I have provided many recipes in chapter 9 to get you started. Because coconut oil is primarily a saturated fat, the heat of cooking does not create a free-radical soup as it does with other vegetable oils. You can feel safe knowing that you aren't damaging your health when you eat it. From all the research that has been done to this point, it appears that coconut oil is the healthiest all-purpose oil you can use.

Coconut oil melts at about 76 degrees F, becoming a clear liquid that looks like almost any other vegetable oil. Below this temperature, it solidifies and takes on a creamy white appearance. At moderate room temperatures it has a soft buttery texture and is sometimes called coconut butter. Coconut oil can be spread on bread as a replacement for butter or margarine. Some brands have a mild, pleasant coconut flavor that makes them excellent spreads. If you like the taste of real butter, you can make a more flavorful spread using half butter and half coconut oil whipped together. Because it has a buttery consistency at normal room temperature, it isn't generally used as a salad dressing. Olive oil, which is a healthy oil when used cold or at room temperature, is better for cold salads. I like to use a mixture of olive and coconut oils for my salads. When coconut oil is mixed with olive oil it remains liquid when poured on a salad.

Coconut oil has a moderately low smoking point, so you need to keep the temperature below 350 degrees F when cooking foods on the stove. This is a moderately high cooking temperature and you can cook anything at this heat, even stir-fry vegetables. If you don't have a temperature gauge on your stovetop, you can tell when it goes over this point because the oil will begin to smoke. When baking breads, muffins, and casseroles using coconut oil, you can set the oven at temperatures above 350 degrees F because the moisture in the food keeps the inside temperature below 212 degrees F.

You don't need any special instructions or recipes to use coconut oil. Simply use it in place of other oils in recipes that call for butter, shortening, margarine, or vegetable oil. Most good brands of coconut oil have a very mild flavor and can be used to cook any type of food. Try it in cookies, cakes, muffins, piecrusts, and pancake batter. It is great for stir-frying or any skillet or stovetop use. Use a melted coconut-butter mixture with seasonings poured over rice, pasta, or vegetables instead of butter or cream sauce.

For frying, nothing beats coconut oil. It isn't absorbed into foods as much as other vegetable oils, doesn't splatter as much, and can be used over again. I don't ordinarily recommend eating fried foods because most vegetable oils become toxic when fried, but if you use coconut oil, fried foods could be good for you, as long as you don't overheat it. Remember to keep the temperature below the point where it starts to smoke. Any oil, including coconut oil, will produce toxic byproducts if overheated.

You can also add coconut oil to most any type of hot beverage such as tea, coffee, hot chocolate, hot cider, eggnog, and even warmed vegetable juice. It tastes good in warm milk and is delicious with V-8 Juice. Prepare the beverage as you normally would and simply stir in a tablespoon or so of coconut oil. The beverage needs to be warm enough to keep the coconut oil in a liquid state (76 degrees or more). Since oil is less dense than water it doesn't mix well with most beverages and tends to rise to the surface. That's okay. Just stir it up and drink. It won't taste oily. This is one of the quickest and easiest ways to add coconut oil to your diet.

Coconut oil is very stable and does not need to be refrigerated. It will stay fresh for at least two or three years unrefrigerated. If kept in a cool place it will last even longer, so it makes a good storage oil. I've heard of coconut oil being analyzed after sitting on the shelf for 15 years and still being unoxidized and safe to use. I buy several jars of oil at a time and keep one in the refrigerator. I do this only because I prefer to use the hardened oil, as opposed to the liquid. To me it's easier to scoop a little out of the jar with a knife or spoon than it is to pour it out. When pouring, it's too easy to spill and drip. If I need liquid oil, all I do is heat up a little in a hot pan, or I will pull the entire jar out of the refrigerator an hour or so before it's needed. It melts quickly.

EATING COCONUTS
AND COCONUT PRODUCTS

Besides pure coconut oil, another source of the oil comes directly from eating the fruit or nut of the seed or from drinking the milk. Fresh coconut meat is about 33 percent oil; 7 ounces of dried coconut provides about 3½ tablespoons of oil. Ten ounces of coconut milk also provides 3½ tablespoons of oil. The more coconut oil you can add to your diet this way, the better. Adding coconut to your recipes can provide a significant amount of this life-giving oil.

DRIED AND FRESH COCONUT

Coconut, both dried and fresh, is a good source of fiber, which is known to be valuable in proper digestive function. One cup of dried, shredded coconut supplies 9 grams of fiber. This is three to four times as much as most fruits and vegetables. For example, broccoli contains only 3 grams of fiber per cup, and raw cabbage has only 2 grams per cup. A cup of white bread has a mere 1 gram. Coconut also contains as much protein as an equal amount of green beans, carrots, and most other vegetables. It contains vitamins B_1, B_2, B_3, B_6, C, and E, folic acid, and the minerals calcium, iron, magnesium, phosphorus, potassium, sodium, and zinc, among others.

Most of the coconut available to us in stores has been dried and shredded. When dried, the moisture content is reduced from 52 percent (in fresh coconut) to about 2.5 percent. The fat content and nutritional content is pretty much the same in dried and fresh coconut. Since the saturated fat is highly resistant to oxidation and spoilage, shredded coconut will last for many months, whereas fresh coconut can spoil in a matter of days.

Fresh coconut is a delight to eat as a snack or to include in your cooking. Most good grocery stores everywhere sell it. You should buy whole coconuts that are as fresh as you can find, but, unfortunately, when you buy a coconut at the store you have no way of telling how old it is. A fresh coconut will stay fresh for many weeks, but an older coconut may be rotten the day you buy it. Shake the shell to detect whether it still contains the water inside. If not, put it back. All three eyes should be intact, and it should not be cracked, leaking, or moldy.

Before opening, you must first drain the liquid. To do this, puncture a hole in at least two of the three eyes with an ice pick. The thin membrane over one of the eyes is relatively soft and easy to pierce. You will easily find that one. The other two eyes require a little more effort to penetrate, and you may need to use a hammer and nail. Once the holes are made, drain the liquid into a glass. After the liquid is removed, you are ready to crack the shell.

Coconut shells are tough and can be very difficult to open. Fresh coconuts straight from the tree have a softer shell and can be opened by a sharp blow with a large knife. But the coconuts sold in most grocery stores are older and have much harder shells. The easiest way to open one of these coconuts is to brace it in a corner and strike it with a hammer. The force to break the shell may be substantial, so choose a corner that will not be harmed. Your kitchen countertop may not be the best place to do this. Cement or hardwood stairs make a good location. You could also use a saw, but this can take a long time.

After the shell is opened, pull the white meat off. A brown, fibrous membrane will be on the side that was in contact with the shell. Peel this off with a vegetable peeler. Your coconut is now ready to eat and enjoy.

Because of its high moisture content, once a coconut has been opened, the coconut and the liquid extracted should be refrigerated and used within a few days to avoid spoiling. The remarkable antimicrobial properties of coconut oil become effective only after it has entered our bodies. Therefore, the oil in the fresh nut will not prevent mold or bacteria growth.

COCONUT MILK

Another common coconut product is coconut milk. Technically speaking coconut milk is *not* the liquid that develops naturally inside the coconut. This liquid is called "coconut water," although the two terms are commonly interchanged. True coconut milk is a manufactured product made from the flesh of the coconut. It is prepared by mixing water with grated coconut, squeezing and extracting the pulp, leaving only the liquid. Coconut milk contains between 17 and 24 percent fat.

The water that fills the cavity inside the coconut is colorless but slightly cloudy and sweet-tasting. Coconut milk, on the other hand, is pure white, resembling cow's milk, and is not sweet unless sugar is added. Canned coconut milk is available in many grocery and health food stores and can be used as a replacement for regular cow's milk and in a wide variety of dishes (see the recipes in chapter 9). You can drink it by the glass, use it in hot and cold cereal, and pour it over fresh fruit. Coconut milk can also be added to many cold beverages. You can combine coconut milk with fruit juice, milk, chocolate milk, and many other cold beverages. Of course, you can mix coconut milk with hot beverages too. One of my favorite drinks is a mixture of coconut milk and orange juice. The coconut milk gives the juice a delicious creamy taste and texture. Mix 2 to 4 tablespoons of coconut milk into 1 cup of orange juice.

You can also use coconut milk to make fruit smoothies, coconut pancakes, clam chowder, and creamy chicken gravy, to mention just a few (see the recipes in chapter 9). With delicious meals like these, dieting can be a pleasure, and because there are no calorie restrictions to worry about, you can easily maintain it for life without feeling hungry or deprived.

APPLYING COCONUT OIL TO YOUR SKIN AND HAIR

Coconut oil works like magic on the skin. Whenever I meet someone who is hesitant about eating coconut oil, I suggest trying it on the skin first and seeing what it does for the skin. Once people begin to use it topically and see the improvement, they become believers and are more willing to add it to their diets. When used as a skin lotion, food-grade coconut oil is preferred. Oil is readily absorbed through the skin and into the body. It's almost the same as eating it. So if you wouldn't eat it, don't put it on your skin.

Because oils are readily absorbed by the skin, another way to get coconut oil into the body is by applying it to the skin. The only problem with skin application is that you can't really tell how much oil is actually absorbed, since absorption varies, depending on skin texture and thickness. In addition, too much oil applied to any one area tends to sit on the surface of the skin, where it is easily rubbed off. Therefore, using coconut oil as a lotion or hair conditioner should not be the only way you incorporate it into your lifestyle. Cooking with coconut oil and eating coconut products will also add luster to your skin and hair. But in order to achieve specific beauty benefits, skin and hair application is recommended.

When we bathe with soap and water, the protective chemical barrier on the skin is washed off, leaving the skin vulnerable to germs that can cause infections. Applying a layer of coconut oil helps to quickly reestablish this barrier. It also lubricates and softens the skin. I recommend you apply a *thin* layer of oil over most of your body. Don't use too much, or it will sit on the surface of the skin and rub off on your clothing. Massage the oil into your skin, focusing on areas where the skin is especially dry, red, infected, cut, or bruised. Working the oil into the skin helps increase absorption and speed healing. Massage the oil on the feet and work it between the toes. This is a great way to prevent and even treat foot fungus. Feet are often abused and neglected, causing them to be dry, cracked, and infected. People often tell me how wonderful their feet look after using coconut oil.

To help control dandruff and improve the appearance of your hair, apply the oil to your scalp and massage it in. Work it into the skin. Let the oil soak into your scalp and hair for a period of time, at least 15 minutes; the longer the better. Then wash it out. If you like, you can apply a small amount of coconut oil to your hair after you get out of the shower. Use only a little. You don't want your hair to look or feel greasy.

Don't be afraid of applying the oil to your face. It will help your complexion. Coconut oil acts like an exfoliant and helps remove dead cells, giving the skin a shiny, youthful appearance.

Coconut oil can help with all types of skin blemishes. I've had deep discolorations caused by injuries that were three or four years old fade away within weeks. Acne outbreaks become less troublesome. Wrinkles, growths, and liver spots start to fade. It soothes and speeds the healing of burns, cuts, insect bites, and other injuries. It keeps skin strong and elastic and is an excellent way to heal stretch marks after childbirth. For best results, the expectant mother should massage the oil into the abdomen every day. This should be continued after delivery until the marks are completely gone.

In chronic conditions, you may or may not see immediate results. The oil aids the body in healing the skin. This usually takes time. Apply it daily, even two or three times a day if necessary. In a matter of weeks you will see the improvement. For best results you should consume the oil as well as apply it to the skin.

WHAT TO DO WHEN YOU ARE SICK

In coastal Africa and South and Central America and other tropical areas of the world, people are known to drink coconut or palm kernel oil whenever they become sick. To them, the tropical oils are both a food and a medicine. Coconut oil can be helpful in fighting many common seasonal illnesses. In the case of a virus, which includes the flu, there is no medication that can destroy the organism. Medications given in these circumstances are primarily to relieve symptoms. The body has to mount its own defense, and you simply must wait it out. Even if you have a bacterial infection and are given antibiotics, your body must still fight off the infection. Whether you have a viral or bacterial infection, you're going to need to eat. You might as well be eating foods prepared in coconut oil. This will provide your body with valuable antimicrobial fatty acids that will aid it in overcoming the illness.

Some people prefer to avoid drugs whenever possible because they don't want the side effects that accompany medications. Coconut oil provides a natural way to fight infection without harmful or unpleasant side effects. Whether you choose to use medications or not, coconut oil can help you fight the infection and get better quicker.

Although there is no standard guideline for what dosage to take when you are sick, I recommend 4–8 tablespoons a day until you feel better. Spread your dosage over the day by taking a couple of tablespoons at each meal. Many people have reported good results overcoming seasonal illnesses by taking a spoonful of oil every couple of hours throughout the day. A large person would need to take more than a smaller person. You can take it by the spoonful if you like, but it is more palatable if you mix it with food. A couple of tablespoons in a glass of orange juice is a quick and easy way to do it. Orange juice, or other beverages, should be at room temperature or warmer to prevent the oil from solidifying. Juice and oil do not mix well, so add the oil, stir, and drink promptly. If this is too much oil for your taste, you can use one of the recipes given in chapter 9. Remember also to get plenty of rest, drink lots of water, and take vitamin supplements, especially vitamin C, to help your body recover. Once you're back to normal, continue to take about 3½ tablespoons (50 grams) of coconut oil daily for maintenance.

If someone is very sick and vomiting, it may not be possible to take coconut oil orally. In this case, you can massage the oil into the skin.

Oils are easily absorbed into the body through the skin. This bypasses the digestive tract, providing the body with needed nourishment, a source of energy, and antimicrobial fatty acids to fight the infection. Even if the infectious organism is not vulnerable to MCFAs, the nourishment the oil provides will strengthen the body, helping it to heal more quickly. I suggest massaging about 1 tablespoon of oil over the entire body two or three times a day. Several thin layers of oil are absorbed much better than one thick layer because too much oil in any one place saturates the tissues and limits absorption, and excess oil often rubs off on clothing and sheets. When applying the oil make sure to massage it into the skin closest to the most infected part of the body. For a sore throat, massage the oil around the neck; for a chest or lung infection, be sure to apply plenty of oil to the chest and back.

The most active antimicrobial ingredient in coconut oil is lauric acid or, more specifically, monolaurin. You can purchase lauric acid in the form of monolaurin as a dietary supplement. This provides a concentrated dose of the most potent germ-fighting fatty acid. It can be taken with a glass of water like any other supplement. This lauric acid supplement, known by the trade name Lauricidin®, is available by mail order (see resources in the appendix). The recommended dose of monolaurin is as follows: at the first sign of infection, take 1,800–3,600 milligrams (6–12 300-mg capsules) daily for four to five days, then taper down to 2–4 capsules until free of symptoms.

Self-diagnosis and treatment may be all right for minor illnesses like a cold; however, I recommend that before treating any serious illness you consult with a physician or other health care provider first. After reading about all the wonderful things coconut oil can do, it's tempting to think of it as a panacea for all illnesses. While coconut oil is good, keep in mind that it's not a cure-all. The MCFAs in coconut oil won't kill all germs, and medical care may be needed.

I think the best use of coconut oil is as a potent nutrient that can help to prevent disease and illness. It is much easier to prevent an illness from developing than it is to cure it once it gets started. If you take 3–4 tablespoons of coconut oil every day and eat a healthy diet, you probably won't get sick. If you do get sick, it will probably be from an infection that is not vulnerable to MCFAs. In this case you may want to use some other natural remedy or standard medication.

A DIETARY CHALLENGE

Scientific knowledge regarding the health benefits of coconut oil began emerging over 40 years ago. Since then its unique health-promoting properties have been recognized by only a small number of researchers. Although products containing coconut oil derivatives have been used to nourish patients in hospitals for many years, the vast majority of doctors, nutritionists, and food scientists have been unaware of its potential health benefits. Consequently, they have often considered coconut oil a source of unhealthy saturated fats that raise blood cholesterol. Fortunately, this is beginning to change as knowledge of the many benefits of coconut oil increases. One of the purposes of this book is to educate the public, as well as health care professionals, about the great potential of coconut oil and to dispel untruths created by the marketing efforts of competitive industries.

Despite the evidence presented in this book, many health care workers and writers will continue to argue and say coconut oil is bad for you. It's hard to accept a new truth when you have been conditioned to believe something else for many years. However, if you have an open mind and are willing to accept new truths, you will welcome the knowledge about coconut oil. There are too many benefits to ignore. I didn't make up this stuff. The information in this book came from published studies and clinical observations as well as historical and epidemiological research. The facts are there, and you can read them yourself if you want to wade through the medical literature (see the references at the end of the book). If you stop to think about it and use a little common sense, it's clear that coconut oil is not harmful. People who consume large quantities of coconuts and coconut oil have been shown to be some of the healthiest on earth. However, you are likely to hear criticism of coconut oil for years to come. But who are you going to believe, the soybean industry and misinformed writers and doctors who are dying right and left from degenerative diseases, or the healthy Pacific Islanders and the researchers making the discoveries? I put my trust in the facts and not the marketing propaganda of the soybean industry.

If naysayers don't want to believe it, don't let that hold you back. You have a great opportunity awaiting you. If you eat coconut oil on a regular basis, the power of these antimicrobial MCFAs will protect your body and support your immune system. Eating coconut oil may provide you with a harmless and inexpensive way of preventing or even fighting off many illnesses. Research may eventually find coconut oil to be just as effective as many of the antimicrobial drugs and vaccines that are currently used. It is definitely safer. Eating coconut oil has no undesirable side effects.

Keep in mind that doctors after graduation from medical school are, for the most part, educated by the pharmaceutical industry. The literature they receive and the seminars they go to are funded almost entirely by these companies. The information they are exposed to is naturally extremely biased, focusing only on drug therapy. For this reason, most doctors know very little about nutrition and even less about current research involving MCFAs. Most doctors will probably be completely ignorant of the research and developments regarding MCFAs for several years to come. They will continue advising you to avoid all saturated fats, including coconut oil, because they don't know any better. They may never have even heard of medium-chain fatty acids or even know that there are many different types of saturated fat. Don't wait for them to catch up with you.

After reading this book, you are armed with knowledge that could greatly enhance your health and improve your quality of life. The simple act of eliminating refined vegetable oils from your diet and replacing them with coconut oil will work wonders for you. You will be replacing a toxic substance with one that offers many marvelous health benefits.

This change should be a lifelong commitment. Eating coconut oil isn't something you should do for only a few months, as so many people do with fad diets. To gain permanent benefit, you need to do it permanently. Ignore the negative comments you may get from others who know nothing about the health benefits of coconut oil. Have them read this book and let them discover the healing miracles of coconut oil for themselves. One of the best presents you can give a friend is the gift of health. Give your friends copies of this book. Not only will you help them gain better health, but you will gain friends who will encourage and support you.

If you still have doubts, I challenge you to try it for six months—just six months, that's all. After six months, see if you don't look and feel better than you did before. My challenge to you is to eliminate all processed vegetable oils from your diet, especially hydrogenated oils (including shortening and margarine). A little butter and extra virgin olive oil is okay. Many people refrain from using butter with the belief that it is bad for them. Milk contains many of the health-promoting MCFAs, including lauric acid. Butter provides a modest source of this important fatty acid. Population studies have shown that when people remove butter from their diets and replace it with margarine their rate of heart disease actually increases! Use coconut oil for all your cooking needs, and use extra virgin olive oil in your salad dressing.

I recommend you start off slowly. Try 1 or 2 *teaspoons* of coconut oil first. Sometimes people take too much and their bodies are not accustomed to handling so much oil, and they experience runny stools. Go slow and gradually build up to about 3 to 4 tablespoons a day. Take the oil with food. Use it in your cooking whenever possible. Add it to foods as you would butter. Use it on your skin.

The hardest thing about this challenge is that if you go out to eat in a restaurant, you often don't know what type of oils they use. If you have a choice, request olive or coconut oil whenever possible. Choose butter over margarine. Otherwise, I suggest you avoid eating in places where you don't know what you're getting. Restaurants are notoriously negligent in regard to customers' health, especially when it comes to oils. They often use the cheapest, degraded, processed oils around. Oils are often heated to very high temperatures repeatedly for days and even weeks at a time, causing them to become extremely rancid and highly toxic. Deep-fried foods such as french fries, chicken nuggets, and donuts are the most toxic foods you can get at a restaurant. If you have to have fried foods, they should be fried in coconut oil because it does not degrade into free radicals or create toxic trans fatty acids when heated, as other vegetable oils do.

Occasionally someone tells me that he or she tried using coconut oil for awhile but didn't see any appreciable improvement. Let me state again that coconut oil is not a cure-all. It will not remedy every health problem. Second, you need to give it a chance. When people tell me it didn't work for them, and I ask them how long they tried it, the answer is three or four days. You cannot expect to see much improvement in just a few days, especially with chronic problems that may have existed for years. Give it a chance. Sometimes it may take weeks or months to see noticeable improvement in conditions that have existed for several years. And the results you get will vary to some degree, depending on your lifestyle choices and diet. If you live on soda pop and donuts, you're not going to experience the same degree of improvement as someone who eats more wisely. Coconut oil aids the body in healing itself. If you don't consume adequate amounts of vitamins and minerals, your body won't be capable of healing, regardless of how much coconut oil you use. That's just common sense.

I know this dietary change will work for you. I've seen it happen in others. I would like to hear from you. Write and tell me how coconut oil has affected your life. You can write to me at The Coconut Research Center, P.O. Box 25203, Colorado Springs, CO 80936. For more information on oils and health, write and ask for a free copy of the *Healthy Ways Newsletter,* or go to the website www.coconutresearchcenter.org.

Your Daily Dose

You could get a daily dose of MCFAs by taking coconut oil the way you would any other liquid dietary supplement—by the spoonful or by mixing it in a beverage. The recommended daily dosage for adults is 3½ tablespoons. Keep in mind that people have achieved good results from eating less oil per day. So if you only eat 1 or 2 tablespoons daily you will still benefit.

Oil, any oil, straight from the spoon is difficult for most people to take. Some people can handle it without a problem, but for most, the oily taste and texture are hard to stomach (figuratively speaking). Virgin coconut oil extracted from fresh coconut milk, however, produces a very delicate flavored product that is so good it can easily be eaten by the spoonful. It is so good it is almost like eating coconut cream. But if eating spoonfuls of oil isn't for you, there are other ways to get the daily dose without having to consume it by the spoonful. Chapter 9 contains a variety of recipes to show how you can get the recommended dose in more palatable ways.

9

RECIPES FOR NUTRITION AND BEAUTY

The recipes in this chapter are useful for people who don't ordinarily use much oil in cooking or food preparation and want to incorporate coconut oil into their diets. Keep in mind that it isn't necessary to take 3½ tablespoons of oil in one single meal; in fact, it's better to spread it out over the entire day. Use these recipes as they are or as examples to create your own and adjust the oil content to suit your needs.

BEVERAGES

Sweetened Coconut Milk

Coconut milk straight from the can is very thick and creamy and not very sweet, which makes it great for use in soups and sauces. Straight from the can it's more like a thick, unsweetened cream and too rich to drink by the glass. With just a little preparation, however, you can make an excellent substitute for cow's milk.

This recipe shows you how to turn a can of coconut milk into a creamy coconut beverage that is good enough to drink by the glass, pour over hot or cold cereal, or combine with freshly cut fruit such as peaches or strawberries in a bowl. Diluting the milk slightly and adding a little honey gives it a mild, pleasant sweetness that will have you wanting to drink it by the glass.

> 1 can (14 oz) coconut milk
> 7 oz water (one-half can)
> 2 tablespoons honey (or other sweetener)
> pinch of salt

- Empty coconut milk into a quart container. Add water, honey, and salt. Mix thoroughly, chill, and serve. *Note:* The honey will dissolve in mixture easily if liquid is at room temperature. For sweeter milk add more honey. For less creamy milk, add more water.
- The recipe makes a little more than 2½ cups milk. Each ½-cup serving of this milk contains approximately 1 tablespoon of coconut oil. A 12-ounce glass (1½ cups) will supply you with approximately 3 tablespoons oil, and 1¾ cups supplies 3½ tablespoons.

MAKES 5 ½-CUP SERVINGS

Flavored Coconut Milk

Vanilla and almond extract give the milk a wonderful added taste. Other extracts may also be added for variety.

2½ cups Sweetened Coconut Milk
1 teaspoon vanilla or almond extract

Simply add the extract to the milk, stir, and serve.

MAKES 5 ½-CUP SERVINGS

BREAKFAST

Hash Browns

Fried potatoes absorb a lot of fat when they are cooked. Coconut oil is an excellent frying fat because of its stability under heat.

1 medium-sized potato
2 tablespoons coconut oil
salt and pepper to taste

Grate the potato and set aside. Heat 2 tablespoons of coconut oil in a frying pan to 300 degrees F. (I use an electric frying pan so I know the exact temperature.) Add the grated potato to the hot pan, spread it out evenly over the bottom of the pan, then push it down with a pancake turner so the potato pieces form a mat. You want the potato to be in contact with the bottom of the pan and the oil.

Cover the pan and cook for about 10–12 minutes. Remove the cover. The potatoes are completely cooked. You do not need to turn the hash browns over and cook the other side. Serve by placing the toasted side up. Season with salt and pepper to taste. One serving (one potato) cooked this way will supply about 2 tablespoons oil.

MAKES 1 SERVING

• • •

Coconut Milk Smoothie

1 ripe banana
1 cup coconut milk
1 cup orange juice

Chill all ingredients before using. Blend all ingredients in a blender until smooth. For a thicker smoothie, you can put it into the freezer for an hour before serving. Contains 2 tablespoons coconut oil per serving.

MAKES 1 SMOOTHIE

• • •

Piña Colada Smoothie

1 cup coconut milk
1 cup orange juice
½ cup fresh chopped pineapple

• Chill all ingredients before using. Blend all ingredients in a blender until smooth. To thicken the smoothie, put it into the freezer for 45 minutes. Contains 2 tablespoons coconut oil per serving.

MAKES 1 SMOOTHIE

* * *

Fruit Smoothie

1 cup coconut milk
1 cup fresh strawberries or blueberries
½ ripe banana
honey (optional)

• Chill ingredients before using. Fruit can be frozen. Blend all ingredients in a blender until smooth. To thicken the smoothie, put it into the freezer for 45 minutes. For a sweeter smoothie, you may add a little honey or other sweetener. Contains 2 tablespoons coconut oil per serving.

MAKES 1 SMOOTHIE

* * *

Fruit Smoothie Blend

1 cup strawberries
1 cup raspberries
1 cup blueberries
1 cup coconut milk

1 cup orange juice

honey (optional)

- Chill ingredients before using. Fruit can be frozen. Blend all ingredients in a blender until smooth. To thicken the smoothie, put it into the freezer for 45 minutes. For a sweeter smoothie, you may add a little honey or other sweetener. Contains 1 tablespoon coconut oil per smoothie.

MAKES 2 SMOOTHIES

• • •

Yogurt Smoothie

You don't always have to use coconut milk to add coconut oil to a smoothie. Here is a recipe that uses coconut oil. The secret to adding coconut oil to a smoothie is to put it in last while the blender is turned on. This way the oil is more evenly dispersed in the drink. If you add coconut oil while mixing the fruit, it tends to harden and form little beads or chunks that some people prefer not to have in a smoothie.

1 cup vanilla yogurt

1 cup fruit juice

2 cups fruit

2 tablespoons melted coconut oil*

- Chill all ingredients except coconut oil before using. Fruit can be frozen. Blend yogurt, juice, and fruit in a blender until smooth. Just before turning off the blender, slowly pour in melted coconut oil.

---

*You may use up to 6 tablespoons of coconut oil if you like. That would give you 3 tablespoons of oil per serving.

Continue to blend for about a minute. Contains 1 tablespoon coconut oil per smoothie.

MAKES 2 SMOOTHIES

• • •

Whole-Wheat Muffins

¾ cup lukewarm water

1 egg

⅓ cup honey

½ cup applesauce

1 teaspoon vanilla

3 tablespoons melted coconut oil

1¾ cups whole-wheat flour

2 teaspoons baking powder

¼ teaspoon salt

Preheat oven to 400 degrees F. Combine water, egg, honey, applesauce, vanilla, and melted coconut oil (not hot) in a bowl and mix thoroughly. In a separate bowl mix together flour, baking powder, and salt. Add the dry ingredients to the liquid, mixing just until moistened. Pour into greased muffin cups. Bake for 15 minutes. Each muffin contains ¼ tablespoon oil. If you increase the coconut oil in the batter to 6 tablespoons, then each muffin will contain ½ tablespoon oil.

MAKES 12 MUFFINS

Blueberry Muffins

This recipe makes delicious whole-wheat blueberry muffins.

½ cup lukewarm water
1 egg
½ cup honey
1 teaspoon vanilla
3 tablespoons melted coconut oil
1½ cups whole-wheat flour
2 teaspoons baking powder
¼ teaspoon salt
1 cup fresh blueberries

- Preheat oven to 400 degrees F. Combine water, egg, honey, vanilla, and melted coconut oil (not hot) in a bowl and mix thoroughly. In a separate bowl mix together flour, baking powder, and salt. Add the dry ingredients to the liquid, mixing just until moistened. Fold in the blueberries. Pour into greased muffin cups. Bake for 15 minutes. Each muffin contains about ¼ tablespoon oil.
- As a variation to this recipe you can substitute another fruit, such as raspberries or cherries, for the blueberries. You can create a variety of delicious muffins using different types of fruits.

MAKES 12 MUFFINS

Coconut Bran Muffins

1 cup water

1 tablespoon vanilla extract

⅓ cup honey

1 egg

¼ cup wheat bran

1 cup whole-wheat flour

¼ cup grated unsweetened coconut

2 teaspoons baking powder

¼ teaspoon salt

1 teaspoon cinnamon

½ teaspoon nutmeg

3 tablespoons melted coconut oil

½ cup nuts

Combine water, vanilla, honey, egg, and bran in a bowl and let sit for about 10 minutes. The bran will absorb some of the moisture as it sits, which will improve the texture of the final product. In another bowl mix flour, coconut, baking powder, salt, cinnamon, and nutmeg. Preheat oven to 400 degrees F. Add melted coconut oil (not hot) to the liquid ingredients, add the nuts, and mix together. Combine the wet and dry ingredients in one bowl and mix just until moist. Do not overmix or the muffins will not rise as well. Pour into greased muffin cups. Bake for 15 minutes. Each muffin contains ¼ tablespoon coconut oil. If you increase the coconut oil in the recipe to 6 tablespoons, each muffin will contain ½ tablespoon oil.

MAKES 12 MUFFINS

Baking-Powder Biscuits

2 cups whole-wheat flour

3 teaspoons baking powder

½ teaspoon salt

5 tablespoons coconut oil

¾ cup coconut milk

Preheat oven to 450 degrees F. Combine flour, baking powder, and salt in a bowl. The coconut oil should be hardened, not melted. Cut coconut oil into flour to form coarse crumbs. Add coconut milk and stir quickly with fork just until dough follows fork around bowl. Knead on lightly floured surface about 10 times. Roll or pat dough to ½-inch thickness. Dip biscuit cutter in flour and cut dough. Place on ungreased cookie sheet and bake for 12 minutes. Each biscuit contains ½ tablespoon coconut oil.

MAKES 10 BISCUITS

• • •

Whole-Wheat Pancakes

¼ cup coconut oil

1½ cups whole-wheat flour

¼ teaspoon salt

2 teaspoons baking powder

1 egg

¾ cup lukewarm water

½ cup applesauce

- Heat coconut oil in skillet over low heat until just melted. Mix flour, salt, and baking powder in a bowl. In a separate bowl, beat egg, water, applesauce, and melted (not hot) oil together. Leave the coconut oil residue in the skillet and increase temperature to moderate heat, about 300 degrees F. As the skillet is heating, combine liquid and dry ingredients and mix only until well dampened. Do not overmix, as this will make pancakes heavier. Use about 3 tablespoons batter for each pancake. Cook until bubbles form over surface, turn gently, and brown the other side. Serve hot with honey, maple syrup, fruit, or other topping.
- Each pancake contains ⅓ tablespoon oil. Three pancakes supply 1 tablespoon oil and six pancakes 2 tablespoons. You can adjust the amount of oil you use. Reducing the amount of coconut oil in the batter to 2 tablespoons would give you 1 tablespoon for every 6 pancakes.

MAKES 12 PANCAKES

• • •

Coconut-Orange Pancakes

1 cup whole-wheat flour

1½ teaspoons baking powder

¼ teaspoon salt

¼ cup grated coconut

1 egg

1 tablespoon molasses

¼ cup coconut oil

1¼ cups lukewarm orange juice

- Mix flour, baking powder, salt, and coconut in a bowl. In a separate bowl, combine egg, molasses, coconut oil, and orange juice. Warm orange juice is used to keep the coconut oil from hardening. Heat an additional tablespoon of coconut oil in a skillet to prevent the pancakes from sticking. Mix the dry ingredients with the wet. Spoon batter onto hot skillet, making pancakes about 2½ to 3 inches in diameter. Serve with your choice of toppings. Each pancake contains ⅓ tablespoon coconut oil.

MAKES ABOUT 12 PANCAKES

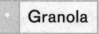

Granola

6 cups old-fashioned oats

2 teaspoons cinnamon

4 cups shredded or flaked coconut

2 cups pecans, chopped

1 cup sunflower seeds

1 cup coconut oil

1 cup honey

1 tablespoon vanilla extract

1 cup raisins

In a large bowl mix together oats, cinnamon, coconut, pecans, and sunflower seeds. Heat oil and honey in a small saucepan over medium heat until just melted, but not hot; remove from heat and add vanilla. Stir honey mixture into oat mixture. Pour into large baking dish. Bake at 325 degrees F for 1 hour and 15 minutes or until oats are golden brown. Stir occasionally while cooking for even browning. Remove from oven and cool. Add raisins. Store in an airtight container. Each serving contains about 1 tablespoon coconut oil.

MAKES 14 1-CUP SERVINGS

Coconut Banana Bread

1 cup coconut oil

2 cups sugar

1 can (5½ ounces) crushed pineapple with juice

4 eggs

1 ripe banana, mashed

4 cups flour

1 cup unsweetened shredded coconut

2 teaspoons baking powder

1 teaspoon baking soda

¾ teaspoon salt

Preheat oven to 350 degrees F. Stir together coconut oil and sugar. Mix in pineapple with juice, eggs, and banana. Add flour, coconut, baking powder, baking soda, and salt. Pour batter into two greased and floured 9" x 5" loaf pans. Bake about 60 minutes, or until knife inserted in the center comes out clean. Loaf can be cut into about 16 ½-inch slices. Each slice contains 1 tablespoon coconut oil.

MAKES 1 LOAF

CONDIMENTS

Seasoned Coconut Oil

A dip popular at some Italian restaurants combines olive oil and seasonings. Bread is dipped into the mixture and eaten as an appetizer. You can make a similar dip using coconut oil in place of olive oil.

3½ tablespoons coconut oil

2 tablespoons onion, finely diced

1 tablespoon garlic, finely diced

½ teaspoon basil

½ teaspoon oregano

¼ teaspoon paprika

¼ teaspoon salt

⅛ teaspoon black pepper (or cayenne pepper)

Combine all ingredients in a small saucepan. Heat until mixture just begins to simmer. Turn off the heat and let sit until cool. Don't overheat; your goal is not to cook it but just help the flavors blend. You can use this as a dip or as a spread for bread, a topping for pasta or vegetables, or a salad dressing.

MAKES ⅓ CUP

• • •

Coconut Mayonnaise

Coconut mayonnaise made with 100 percent coconut oil, as in this recipe, tastes best when it is freshly made. When it is refrigerated it tends to harden because the oil solidifies. If you have mayonnaise left over after making this recipe and intend to use it a day or two later, bring it out of the refrigerator and let it sit at room temperature for about 30 minutes before using (depending on how warm your kitchen is). This will allow time for it to soften. The texture won't be as good as when it was freshly made, but it will still be usable.

1 egg

1 tablespoon apple cider vinegar

½ tablespoon prepared mustard

⅛ teaspoon paprika

¼ teaspoon salt

1¼ cups melted coconut oil

Combine egg, vinegar, mustard, paprika, salt, and ¼ cup of melted (not hot) coconut oil in blender or food processor. Blend for about 60 seconds. While machine is running, pour in the remaining coconut oil *very* slowly in a fine, steady stream. The secret to making good mayonnaise is to add the oil in *slowly*. Mayonnaise will thicken as oil is added. Taste and adjust seasoning as needed. Each tablespoon of mayonnaise will contain about ½ tablespoon of coconut oil.

MAKES 1½ CUPS

• • •

Vinegar and Oil Dressing

One of the drawbacks to using coconut oil as a salad dressing is its high melting point (76 degrees). Salads are usually served chilled, so when coconut oil is added, it hardens. You can get around this characteristic if you mix coconut oil with another oil that has a lower melting point, such as olive oil. This recipe is a good example.

¼ cup coconut oil

¼ cup extra virgin olive oil

3 tablespoons water

¼ cup apple cider vinegar

½ teaspoon salt

⅛ teaspoon black pepper

- Put all ingredients into a screw-top jar. Cover and shake vigorously until well blended. Let stand at room temperature for 1 hour. Store in the refrigerator. The oil will eventually rise to the top and harden in the refrigerator. It will melt if you set it out at room temperature for an hour or so. You may also speed the melting of the oil by submerging the jar in hot water for a few minutes. Each tablespoon of dressing contains about ¼ tablespoon of coconut oil.

MAKES 1 CUP

• • •

Buttermilk Dressing

¾ cup Coconut Mayonnaise (page 192)
½ cup buttermilk
1 teaspoon dried dill
½ teaspoon onion powder
¼ teaspoon garlic powder
½ teaspoon salt
dash of black pepper

- Blend all ingredients together. Refrigerate for at least 1 hour. Each tablespoon of dressing contains about ⅓ tablespoon coconut oil.

MAKES 1 CUP

SALADS

Tomato Vinaigrette Salad

2 medium tomatoes, sliced

lettuce leaves

¾ cup Vinegar and Oil Dressing (page 193)

1 teaspoon oregano

½ teaspoon salt

¼ teaspoon pepper

¼ teaspoon dry mustard

1 clove garlic, crushed

4 scallions, finely chopped

1 tablespoon finely chopped cilantro

On each serving plate lay tomato slices on top of a bed of lettuce leaves. Mix together Vinegar and Oil Dressing, oregano, salt, pepper, mustard, and garlic and pour over tomatoes. Garnish with scallions and cilantro. Each serving contains ¾ tablespoon of coconut oil.

SERVES 4

Waldorf Salad

4 medium-sized tart apples, diced

¾ cup finely chopped celery

⅓ cup walnuts, chopped

½ cup raisins

¾ cup Coconut Mayonnaise (page 192)

lettuce leaves

Mix all ingredients together. Serve on a bed of lettuce leaves. Each serving contains 1½ tablespoons coconut oil.

SERVES 4

• • •

Fruit and Coconut Salad

1½ cups chopped fresh pineapple

2 bananas, sliced

2 oranges, peeled and diced

2 apples, cored and diced

1 cup raisins or chopped dates

½ cup shredded coconut

¾ cup Coconut Mayonnaise (page 192)

lettuce leaves

Mix all ingredients together. Serve on bed of lettuce leaves. Each serving contains 1 tablespoon coconut oil.

SERVES 6

Potato Salad

2 pounds (about 6 medium-sized) red potatoes

1 small onion, chopped

½ cup finely chopped dill pickle

¼ cup Vinegar and Oil Dressing (page 193)

1 teaspoon salt

⅛ teaspoon pepper

½ cup Coconut Mayonnaise (page 192)

1 medium stalk celery, chopped

2 hard-boiled eggs, coarsely chopped

Chop potatoes into ½-inch cubes and cook in boiling water until tender. Drain water and let cool. Mix potatoes with the rest of the ingredients, cover, and chill slightly before serving. Each serving contains ½ tablespoon coconut oil.

SERVES 4

• • •

Three-Bean Salad

1 can (16 oz) green beans

1 can (16 oz) wax beans

1 can (16 oz) red kidney beans

1 cup chopped celery

4 scallions, finely chopped

1 cup chopped bell pepper

½ cup chopped dill pickle

¾ cup Vinegar and Oil Dressing (page 193)
½ teaspoon salt
⅛ teaspoon black pepper

• Mix all ingredients. Chill briefly and serve. Each serving contains ½ tablespoon coconut oil.

SERVES 6

• • •

Tomato and Garbanzo Bean Salad

2 medium tomatoes, chopped
½ cup finely chopped bell pepper
½ cup chopped Bermuda or Spanish onion
1 clove garlic, crushed
1 can (16 oz) garbanzo beans, drained
¼ cup minced cilantro
½ teaspoon dried marjoram or oregano
¼ teaspoon salt
⅛ teaspoon black pepper
½ cup Vinegar and Oil Dressing (page 193)

• Put all ingredients in a large bowl and mix well. Cover and let sit at room temperature at least 1 hour. Toss well before serving. Contains ½ tablespoon coconut oil per serving.

SERVES 4

Macaroni Salad

½ pound elbow macaroni

1 cup diced celery

½ cup diced scallions

⅓ cup finely chopped bell pepper

1 cup Coconut Mayonnaise (page 192)

2 tablespoons white vinegar or lemon juice

2 teaspoons prepared mustard

1½ teaspoons salt

⅛ teaspoon black pepper

Cook macaroni according to package directions, drain, and chill. Combine macaroni with remaining ingredients, cover, and chill briefly before serving. Each serving contains 2 tablespoons coconut oil.

SERVES 4

VARIATION: Add 3 cups cubed cooked chicken and an extra ⅓ cup mayonnaise. Can be served as an entrée. Makes 6 servings. Each serving contains approximately 2 tablespoons coconut oil.

SOUPS

Clam Chowder

½ cup water

1 bottle (8 oz) clam juice

½ cup minced yellow onion

4 cloves garlic, minced

1 stalk celery, chopped

2 cups diced potatoes

1 teaspoon salt

⅛ teaspoon white pepper

1 can (14 oz) coconut milk

1 can (8 oz) minced or chopped clams

¼ teaspoon paprika

In a medium saucepan heat water, clam juice, onion, garlic, celery, potatoes, salt, and pepper to boiling. Reduce heat and simmer for about 20 minutes or until potatoes are tender. Add coconut milk and clams with their liquid. Cook for about 5 minutes until heated through. Sprinkle with paprika. Each serving contains 1 tablespoon coconut oil. You may easily increase the amount of coconut oil in this dish by simply adding it.

SERVES 4

Cream of Asparagus Soup

1 pound asparagus, washed, trimmed, and cut in 1-inch pieces

½ cup chopped celery

¼ cup chopped onion

1 cup water

1 can (14 oz) coconut milk

1¼ teaspoon salt

⅛ teaspoon pepper

¼ teaspoon tarragon

Simmer asparagus, celery, and onion in water for 20 minutes or until very tender. Add coconut milk. Puree, a little at a time, in an electric blender at low speed. Return to pan and add salt, pepper, and tarragon, stirring occasionally, until hot but not boiling. Each serving contains 1⅓ teaspoons coconut oil.

SERVES 3

• • •

Cream of Artichoke Soup

½ cup chopped celery

¼ cup chopped onion

2 cloves garlic

2 tablespoons coconut oil

2 tablespoons flour

1 cup water

1 can (14 oz) coconut milk

1 can (14 oz) artichoke hearts, drained and rinsed

1 teaspoon salt

¼ teaspoon white pepper

¼ teaspoon thyme

• Sauté celery, onion, and garlic in coconut oil in a heavy saucepan over low heat until vegetables are tender. Stir in flour and cook for 2 minutes. Add water and coconut milk and bring to a boil. Reduce heat and simmer for 8 to 10 minutes. Puree half the mixture and all of the artichoke hearts in an electric blender; add to pan. Add remaining ingredients and heat, stirring, 2 to 3 minutes. Each serving contains 2 tablespoons coconut oil. You can increase or decrease the oil content by adjusting the amount of oil used to sauté the vegetables.

SERVES 3

• • •

Cream of Cauliflower Soup

2 cups chopped cauliflower

½ cup chopped celery

½ cup chopped onion

1 cup water

2 tablespoons butter

2 tablespoons flour

1 can (14 oz) coconut milk

1¼ teaspoon salt

⅛ teaspoon black pepper

¼ teaspoon curry powder

• Simmer cauliflower, celery, and onion in water for 20 minutes or until very tender. Puree, a little at a time, in an electric blender at low speed. Heat butter in a saucepan over medium heat; blend in flour and cook until lightly browned, stirring frequently. Add coconut milk slowly, stirring until smooth. Mix in puree, salt, pepper, and curry powder, stirring occasionally, until hot but not boiling. Contains 1⅓ tablespoons coconut oil per serving.

SERVES 3

• • •

Vegetable Beef Stew

Coconut oil can easily be added to many of your favorite dishes. This recipe shows you how simple it can be.

¼ cup coconut oil

1 pound beef, cut into bite-size pieces

½ onion, chopped

2 carrots, chopped

3 cups water

½ cup tomato sauce

2 medium potatoes, chopped*

1 cup green beans

1 tablespoon diced cilantro

salt and pepper

Heat coconut oil in a large saucepan over medium heat. Add beef and lightly brown. Add onion and carrots and cook until tender, stirring frequently. Add water, tomato sauce, potatoes, and green beans; cover and simmer for 20 minutes or until vegetables are tender. Add cilantro and salt and pepper to taste and cook 1 additional

*For a low-carb vegetable beef stew, replace potatoes with 2 cups chopped cauliflower.

minute. Each serving contains 1 tablespoon coconut oil. You may adjust the oil content by adding more or less.

SERVES 4

ENTRÉES

Chicken Salad

3 cups diced cooked chicken

1 cup diced celery

¼ cup minced Bermuda or Spanish onion

¼ cup minced bell pepper

2 tablespoons pimiento

¾ cup Coconut Mayonnaise (page 192)

2 tablespoons lemon juice

¼ teaspoon salt

⅛ teaspoon black pepper

paprika

Mix all ingredients, except paprika, together, cover, and chill briefly before serving. Garnish with paprika before serving. Each serving contains 1 tablespoon coconut oil.

SERVES 6

Egg Salad

12 hard-boiled eggs, chilled, coarsely chopped
1 tablespoon minced yellow onion
½ cup minced celery
1 tablespoon minced parsley
1 teaspoon salt
⅛ teaspoon black pepper
⅓ cup Coconut Mayonnaise (page 192)

Mix all ingredients together. Stir well and serve on a bed of lettuce, on sliced tomatoes, or as a sandwich spread. Each serving contains ¾ tablespoon coconut oil.

SERVES 4

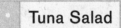

Tuna Salad

2 cans (7 oz each) tuna, drained and flaked
½ cup minced Bermuda onion
juice of ½ lemon
½ cup Coconut Mayonnaise (page 192)
2 tablespoons minced cilantro
½ teaspoon dried dill
dash of salt
⅛ teaspoon black pepper

- Mix all ingredients together. Serve on a bed of lettuce leaves or sliced tomatoes. May also be used as a sandwich spread. Each serving contains 1 tablespoon coconut oil.

SERVES 4

• • •

Curried Shrimp Salad

⅓ cup Coconut Mayonnaise (page 192)

3 tablespoons sour cream

1 teaspoon curry powder

1 teaspoon lemon juice

2 scallions, minced

⅛ teaspoon black pepper

1 pound shrimp, cooked and shelled

mixed lettuce leaves

- Mix all ingredients, except lettuce, together. Serve on a bed of mixed lettuce leaves. Each serving contains ¾ tablespoon coconut oil.

SERVES 4

• • •

Chicken Oriental

¼ cup coconut oil

1 medium onion, chopped

3 cloves garlic, chopped

½ bell pepper, chopped

½ head broccoli, sliced

1 pound chicken, cut in bite-sized pieces

8 ounces mushrooms, sliced

2 cups bean sprouts

1 teaspoon ground ginger

1 teaspoon salt

3 tablespoons cornstarch

1½ cups chicken broth or water

¼ cup tamari sauce

½ cup sliced almonds, toasted

· Heat coconut oil in large skillet over medium heat. Add onion, garlic, bell pepper, and broccoli and sauté until tender. Add chicken, mushrooms, bean sprouts, ginger, and salt; cover and cook, stirring occasionally, for about 3 minutes. Mix cornstarch into chicken broth and add to skillet, stirring constantly, until thick and bubbly. Remove from heat. Stir in tamari sauce. Serve topped with toasted almonds. Each serving contains 1 tablespoon coconut oil.

SERVES 4

• • •

Broccoli Smothered in Coconut Chicken Sauce

1 large head broccoli divided into flowerets (about 4 cups)

½ cup chopped green pepper

½ onion, chopped (about ½ cup)

¼ cup coconut oil

¼ cup flour

1 teaspoon salt

¼ teaspoon pepper

1 can (14 oz) coconut milk

1 cup water or chicken broth

1 can (4 oz) mushroom stems and pieces, drained

3 cups cut-up cooked chicken

- Cook broccoli in steamer. While broccoli is cooking, sauté green pepper and onion in coconut oil over medium heat for 5 minutes; remove from heat. Blend in flour, salt, and pepper. Cook over low heat, stirring constantly, until vegetables are tender; remove from heat. Stir in coconut milk, water, mushrooms, and chicken. Heat to boiling, stirring frequently; reduce heat and simmer for about 10 minutes, until sauce thickens. Serve over hot steamed broccoli. Each serving contains 1 tablespoon coconut oil.

SERVES 4

• • •

Salmon in Coconut Cream Sauce

1 can (14 oz) coconut milk

1 tablespoon cornstarch

1 teaspoon curry powder

⅛ teaspoon salt

⅛ teaspoon white pepper

1 to 1½ pounds salmon fillets, skinned

½ cup chopped tomato

¼ cup fresh chopped cilantro

- Preheat oven to 350 degrees F. In a casserole dish mix coconut milk, cornstarch, curry, salt, and pepper. Add salmon, cover, and bake for 1 hour. Serve salmon covered with the cream sauce and topped with fresh tomato and cilantro. Goes well with a little of the sauce poured on a side dish of vegetables such as broccoli, green beans, or peas. Each serving contains 1 tablespoon coconut oil. More oil may be added if desired.

SERVES 4

• • •

Fillet of Sole in Coconut Milk

¼ cup coconut oil

1 onion, chopped

1 bell pepper, chopped

2 cups chopped cauliflower

5 cloves garlic, chopped

4 sole fillets*

1 teaspoon cornstarch

1 teaspoon garam masala†

1 can (14 oz) coconut milk

salt and black pepper, to taste

Heat coconut oil in skillet and sauté onion, pepper, cauliflower, and garlic until tender. Push vegetables to side of skillet and add sole. Stir cornstarch and garam masala into coconut milk and add to skillet. Cover and simmer for 10 minutes. Add salt and pepper. Contains 2 tablespoons coconut oil per serving.

SERVES 4

---

*You may use any type of white fish in this recipe.

†Garam masala is a blend of spices commonly used in Indian cuisine and similar to curry powder. It's available in the spice section of most grocery stores. If you don't have garam masala, you can use curry powder.

Thai Shrimp and Noodles

8 to 10 oz wheat or rice noodles
¼ cup coconut oil
1 onion, chopped
1 green pepper, chopped
1 head broccoli, chopped
1 teaspoon green curry paste*
½ pound shrimp, peeled, tails off
¼ cup fish sauce*
salt to taste

- Cook noodles according to package directions. Heat coconut oil in a skillet and sauté onion, green pepper, and broccoli until tender. Add green curry paste and shrimp and continue cooking for 5 minutes or until shrimp is cooked. Add fish sauce, remove from heat, and stir in noodles. Add salt to taste. Each serving contains 1 tablespoon coconut oil.

SERVES 4

---

* Green curry paste and fish sauce are popular flavorings used in Thai cooking. You can find them in the Asian section of the grocery store.

DESERTS

Whole-Wheat Coconut Brownies

½ cup coconut oil

2 eggs

1 cup sugar

1 teaspoon vanilla extract

¾ cup whole-wheat flour

⅓ cup cocoa powder

½ teaspoon baking powder

¼ teaspoon salt

½ cup pecans, chopped

1 cup shredded or flaked coconut

Preheat oven to 350 degrees F. Blend coconut oil and eggs together. Mix in sugar and vanilla and set aside. In a separate bowl mix flour, cocoa, baking powder, and salt. Mix together wet and dry ingredients. Stir in pecans. Pour batter into a greased 8" x 8" x 2" baking dish. Sprinkle coconut on top and bake 30 to 35 minutes. Cool to room temperature and cut into 16 squares. Each square contains ½ tablespoon coconut oil.

MAKES 16 SQUARES

Coconut Cookies

3 cups flour

1½ cups grated or shredded coconut

1½ teaspoons baking powder

1 teaspoon salt

1¼ cups coconut oil

3 eggs

1½ cups sugar

1½ teaspoons almond extract

Preheat oven to 375 degrees F. Mix together flour, coconut, baking powder, and salt and set aside. Blend coconut oil, eggs, sugar, and almond extract. Mix wet and dry ingredients together. Roll dough into 1½-inch balls and place 2 inches apart on cookie sheet. Flatten balls to about ½-inch thickness. Bake for 12 to 15 minutes, until pale tan. Transfer to wire racks to cool. Each cookie contains ½ tablespoon coconut oil.

MAKES 36 TO 40 COOKIES

• • •

Coconut Oatmeal Cookies

1 cup brown sugar

½ cup coconut oil

2 eggs

½ teaspoon vanilla extract

1½ cups flour

1 cup oats

½ cup shredded or grated coconut

½ teaspoon baking soda

½ teaspoon cinnamon

¼ teaspoon salt

½ cup walnuts, chopped

Preheat oven to 375 degrees F. Mix together sugar, coconut oil, eggs, and vanilla. In a separate bowl, combine flour, oats, coconut, baking soda, cinnamon, and salt; stir into wet mixture. Fold in walnuts. Roll into 1½-inch balls and place on ungreased cookie sheet 2 inches apart and slightly flatten. Bake for 15 minutes. Each cookie contains ⅓ tablespoon coconut oil.

MAKES 24 COOKIES

• • •

Whole-Wheat Coconut Cake

2⅓ cups whole-wheat flour

1⅔ cups sugar

1¼ teaspoons baking powder

1 teaspoon baking soda

1 teaspoon salt

1 cup coconut oil

2 eggs

2 ripe bananas, mashed

2 teaspoons lemon juice

¾ cups walnuts, chopped

1 cup shredded coconut

Preheat oven to 350 degrees F. Mix flour, sugar, baking powder, baking soda, and salt in large mixing bowl. Add coconut oil, eggs, bananas, and lemon juice and mix until all flour is dampened. Beat vigorously 2 minutes. Fold in walnuts. Sprinkle top with coconut. Bake in a greased and lightly floured 13" x 9" x 2" pan for 35 minutes or until knife inserted in center comes out clean. Cool 10 minutes in pan. Cut into slices. Each slice contains 1 tablespoon coconut oil.

MAKES 16 PIECES

● RESOURCES

For additional information about the health and dietary aspects of fats and oils, particularly coconut oil and medium-chain fatty acids, refer to the resources listed here. If you can't find these books at your local bookstore, they are available from their publishers or from Amazon.com.

BOOKS

Bruce Fife, N.D. *Coconut Lover's Cookbook.* Piccadilly Books, 2004. (719) 550-9887. An entire book devoted to coconut cuisine. Contains 450 recipes using coconut products.

Bruce Fife, N.D. *Eat Fat, Look Thin: A Safe and Natural Way to Lose Weight Permanently.* Piccadilly Books, 2002. (719) 550-9887. Fat can be good for you and can help you lose unwanted weight—if it's the right kind of fat. This book explains the "Coconut Diet," which will help you shed excess weight without counting calories or giving up favorite foods. Includes recipes.

Charles T. McGee, M.D. *Heart Frauds: Uncovering the Biggest Health Scam in History.* Piccadilly Books, 2001. (719) 550-9887. The cholesterol theory of heart disease was disproved years ago, yet everyone is paranoid about cholesterol levels. The medical, pharmaceutical, and food industries continue to promote the cholesterol myth, all for the sake of profit. This book reveals the history of the cholesterol theory and explains why the medical profession is so reluctant to abandon it. For the sake of your health, you should read this revealing book.

Sally Fallon, Mary G. Enig, Ph.D., and Patricia Connolly. *Nourishing Traditions: The Cookbook That Challenges Politically Correct Nutrition and the Diet Dictorats.* New Trends, 1999. (877) 707-1776. More than just a cookbook, this book is about eating the kinds of real food that have nourished people all over the world for centuries. It combines the wisdom of the ancients with the latest accurate scientific research. Contains insights from a variety of doctors and nutritionists. Great recipes that include healthy oils like coconut oil.

Mary G. Enig, Ph.D. *Know Your Fats: The Complete Primer for Understanding the Nutrition of Fats, Oils, and Cholesterol.* Bethesda Press, 2000. (301) 680-8600. An accurate overview of the health aspects of various fats and oils, including the benefits of coconut oil.

WEBSITES

www.coconutresearchcenter.org
This is the website for the Coconut Research Center, the premier source for accurate information on the health and nutritional aspects of coconut products. The website contains news and articles on the health aspects of coconut and provides many helpful resources, including links to other related websites.

www.lauric.org
The Center for Research on Lauric Oils, Inc., maintains this website summarizing recent research in lauric and capric acids. Contains some very interesting information and links to other websites.

www.price-pottenger.org
The Price-Pottenger Nutrition Foundation promotes principles of sound nutrition based on the discoveries and work of Weston A. Price, D.D.S., and Francis M. Pottenger, Jr., M.D.

www.westonaprice.org
This is an excellent resource for dietary and nutritional information, sponsored by the Weston A. Price Foundation, which is dedicated to educating the public about the facts regarding diet and nutrition and dispelling myths perpetuated by commercial enterprises. This site contains lots of excellent articles on a variety of nutritional topics, including coconut and other oils.

PRODUCTS

Most grocery stores carry coconut milk, shredded coconut, and fresh coconuts. Coconut oil, however, is a little more difficult to find. The best place to find coconut oil is in a health food store. If your local store doesn't stock it, ask them to order it. If you can't get a good-quality coconut oil in your area, you can order directly from the distributors listed here or search the Internet under "coconut" or "coconut oil." The companies listed here sell a variety of coconut products, including dietary supplements, soaps, and lotions. Call or check out their websites for the types of products they sell.

BODY FRIENDLY PROVISIONS
52 Riley Road, No. 180
Celebration, FL 34747
(888) 769-0754
www.bodyfriendlyprovisions.com.

CAROTEC, INC.
P.O. Box 9919
Naples, FL 34101-1919
(800) 522-4279
www.carotecinc.com

COCONUT CONNECTIONS
5 Sycamore Dene
Chesham, Bucks
HP5 3JT
UK
01494 771419
www.coconut-connections.com

COCONUT OIL ONLINE
1531 E. Main Street
Eaton, OH 45320
(800) 922-1744
www.coconutoil-online.com

COCONUT OIL UK
P.O. Box 11045
Dickens Health, Solihull
B90 12D
UK
01217 445753
www.coconut-oil-uk.com

CREATION'S BEST
N68W33290 Cty Road K
Oconomowoc, WI 53066
(719) 596-4875
www.creationsbest.com

DR. LaMAR'S HEALTH PRODUCTS
2800 W. 6th Avenue
Emporia, KS 66801
(620) 343-8222
www.drlamarsproducts.com

GRAIN AND SALT SOCIETY
273 Fairway Drive
Asheville, NC 28805
(800) 867-7258
www.celtic-seasalt.com

MT. MAYON LIVING PRODUCTS
8 Klee Court
East Windsor, NJ 08520
(201) 920-5498
www.mtmayon.com

NATURESECRETS AG
Industriestr. 12
CH-8212
Neuhausen, Switzerland
0041-52-670-0161 (Switzerland)
0049-7121-677-283 (Germany)
www.naturesecrets.com

NUTIVA
P.O. Box 1716
Sebastopol, CA 95473
(800) 993-4367
www.nutiva.com

OMEGA NUTRITION, USA
6515 Aldrich Road
Bellingham, WA 98226
(800) 661-3529
www.omegahealthstore.com

QUALITY FIRST INTERNATIONAL INC.
6852 Wellington Road, No. 34
R.R. 22
Cambridge, ON
N3C 2V4
Canada
(877) 441-9479
www.qualityfirst.on.ca.

RADIANT LIFE
P.O. Box 2326
Novato, CA 94948
(888) 593-8333
www.radiantlifecatalog.com

SIMPLY COCONUT
4164 Austin Bluffs Pkwy.
Suite 184
Colorado Springs, CO 80918
(719) 596-4875
www.simplycoconut.com

TROPICAL TRADITIONS, INC.
PMB 219–823 S. Main Street
West Bend, WI 53095
(866) 311-2626
www.tropicaltraditions.com

WILDERNESS FAMILY NATURALS
511 Wisconsin Drive
New Richmond, WI 54017
(866) 936-6457
www.wildernessfamilynaturals.com

• REFERENCES

CHAPTER 1 • THE TRUTH ABOUT COCONUT OIL

Blonz, E. R. Scientists revising villain status of coconut oil. *Oakland Tribune,* January 23, 1991.

Enig, M. G. 1999. Coconut: In support of good health in the twenty-first century. Paper presented at the Thirty-sixth Annual Meeting of the APCC.

Enig, M. G. 2000. *Know your fats.* Silver Spring, Md.: Bethesda Press.

Heimlich, J. 1990. *What your doctor won't tell you.* New York: Harper Perennial.

Konlee, M. 1997. Return from the jungle: An interview with Chris Dafoe. *Positive Health News* 14 (summer).

Okoji, G. O., Peterside I. E., Oruamabo R. S., 1993. Childhood convulsions: A hospital survey on traditional remedies. *African Journal of Medicine and Medical Sciences* 22(2).

Price, W. A. 1998. *Nutrition and physical degeneration.* 6th ed. Los Angeles: Keats.

Prior, I. A. M. 1971. The price of civilization. *Nutrition Today,* July/August.

Spencer, P. L. 1995. Fat faddists. *Consumers' Research* 78(5).

CHAPTER 2 • UNDERSTANDING FATS

Addis, P. B., and G. J. Warner. 1991. In *Free radicals and food additives,* edited by O. I. Aruoma and B. Halliwell. London: Taylor and Francis.

Ball, M. J. 1993. Parenteral nutrition in the critically ill: Use of a medium chain triglyceride emulsion. *Intensive Care Medicine* 19(2).

Belitz, H. D., and W. Grosch. 1999. *Food chemistry.* 2nd ed. Translated by D. Hadziyev. New York: Springer-Verlag.

Booyens, J., and C. C. Louwrens. 1986. "The Eskimo diet: Prophylactic effects ascribed to the balanced presence of natural cis unsaturated fatty acids. *Medical Hypotheses* 21.

Calabrese, C., Myer S., Munson S., Turet P., Birdsall T. C. 1999. A cross-over study of the effect of a single oral feeding of medium chain triglyceride oil vs. canola oil on post-ingestion plasma triglyceride levels in healthy men. *Alternative Medicine Review.* 4(1).

Carroll, K. K., and H. T. Khor. 1971. Effects of level and type of dietary fat on incidence of mammary tumors induced in female Sprague-Dawley rates by 7, 12-dimethylbenzanthracene. *Lipids* 6.

Jiang, Z. M., Zhang S. Y., Wang X. R. 1993. A comparison of medium-chain and long-chain triglycerides in surgical patients. *Annals of Surgery* 217(2).

Kritchevsky, D., and S. A. Pepper. 1967. Chlolesterol vehicle in experimental atherosclerosis. 9. Comparison of heated corn oil and heated olive oil. *Journal of Atherosclerosis Research* 7.

Loliger, J. 1991. In *Free radicals and food additives,* edited by O. I. Aruoma and B. Halliwell. London: Taylor and Francis.

McCully, K. S. 1997. *The homocysteine revolution.* Los Angeles: Keats.

Moore, T. H. 1989. The cholesterol myth. *Atlantic Monthly,* September.

Passwater, R. A. 1985. *The antioxidants.* New Canaan, Conn.: Keats.

Passwater, R. A. 1992. *The new superantioxidant-plus.* New Canaan, Conn.: Keats.

Raloff, J. 1996. Unusual fats lose heart-friendly image. *Science News* 150(6).

Tantibhedhyangkul, P., and S. A. Hashim. 1978. Medium-chain triglyceride feeding in premature infants: Effects on calcium and magnesium absorption. *Pediatrics* 61(4).

Thampan, P. K. 1994. *Facts and fallacies about coconut oil.* Jakarta: Asian and Pacific Coconut Community.

Willett, W. C., Stampfer M. J., Manson J. E., Colditz G. A., Speizer F. E., Rosner B. A., Sampson L. A., Hennekens C. H. 1993. Intake of trans fatty acids and risk of coronary heart disease among women. *Lancet* 341(8845).

CHAPTER 3 • A NEW WEAPON AGAINST HEART DISEASE

Anonymous. 1998. Bad teeth and gums a risk factor for heart disease? *Harvard Heart Letter* 9(3).

Ascherio, A., and W. C. Willett. 1997. Health effects of trans fatty acids. *American Journal of Clinical Nutrition* 66(4 supp.).

Baba, N. 1982. Enhanced thermogenesis and diminished deposition of fat in response to overfeeding with a diet containing medium chain triglycerides. *American Journal of Clinical Nutrition* 35.

Bray, G. A., Cee M., Bray T. L. 1980. Weight gain of rats fed medium-chain triglycerides is less than rats fed long-chain triglycerides. *International Journal of Obesity* 4.

Danesh, J., and R. Collins. 1997. Chronic infections and coronary heart disease: Is there a link? *Lancet* 350.

Enig, M. G. 1993. Diet, serum cholesterol and coronary heart disease. In *Coronary heart disease: The dietary sense and nonsense,* edited by G. V. Man. London: Janus.

Enig, M. G. 1999. Coconut: In support of good health in the twenty-first century. Paper presented at the Thirty-sixth Annual Meeting of the APCC.

Enig, M. G. 2000. *Know your fats: The complete primer for understanding the nutrition of fats, oils, and cholesterol.* Silver Spring, Md.: Bethesda Press.

Fong, I. W. 2000. Emerging relations between infectious diseases and coronary artery disease and atherosclerosis. *Canadian Medical Association Journal* 163(1).

Gaydos, C. A., Summersgill J. T., Sahney N. N., Ramirez J. A., Quinn, T. C. 1996. Replication of Chlamydia pneumoniae in vitro in human macrophages, endothelial cells, and aortic artery smooth muscle cells. *Infection and Immunity* 64.

Geliebter, A. 1983. Overfeeding with medium-chain triglycerides diet results in diminished deposition of fat. *American Journal of Clinical Nutrition* 37.

Greenberger, N. J., and T. G. Skillman. 1969. Medium-chain triglycerides: physiologic considerations and clinical implications. *New England Journal of Medicine* 280.

Gura, T. 1998. Infections: A cause of artery-clogging plaques? *Science* 281.

Hegsted, D. M., McGandy R. B., Myers M. L., Stare F. J. 1965. Qualitative effects of dietary fat on serum cholesterol in man. *American Journal of Clinical Nutrition* 17.

Heimlich, J. 1990. *What your doctor won't tell you.* New York: HarperCollins.

Hornung, B., Amtmann E., Sauer G. 1994. Lauric acid inhibits the maturation of vesicular stomatitis virus. *Journal of General Virology* 75.

Kaunitz, H. 1986. Medium chain triglycerides (MCT) in aging and arteriosclerosis. *Journal of Environmental Pathology, Toxicology, and Oncology* 6 (3-4).

Kaunitz, H., and C. S. Dayrit. 1992. Coconut oil consumption and coronary heart disease. *Philippine Journal of Internal Medicine* 30.

Kurup, P. A., and T. Rajmohan. 1994. Consumption of coconut oil and coconut kernel and the incidence of atherosclerosis. In *Coconut and Coconut Oil in Human Nutrition, Proceedings.* Symposium on Coconut and Coconut Oil in Human Nutrition, sponsored by the Coconut Development Board, Kochi, India, March 27, 1994.

Leinonen, M. 1993. Pathogenic mechanisms and epidemiology of Chlamydia pneumoniae. *European Heart Journal* 14(supp. K).

Mendis, S., and R. Kumarasunderam. 1990. The effect of daily consumption of coconut fat and soya-bean fat on plasma lipids and lipoproteins of young normolipidaemic men. *British Journal of Nutrition* 63.

Millman, C. 1999. The route of all evil. *Men's Health* 14(10).

Muhlestein, J. B. 2003. Chronic infection and coronary artery disease. *Clinical Cardiology* 21(3).

Price, W. A. 1998. *Nutrition and physical degeneration*. 6th ed. Los Angeles: Keats.

Prior, I. A., Davidson F., Salmond C. E., Czochanska Z. 1981. Cholesterol, coconuts, and diet on Polynesian atolls: A natural experiment: The Pukapuka and Tokelau Island studies. *American Journal of Clinical Nutrition* 34(8).

Ross, R. 1993. The pathogenesis of atherosclerosis: A perspective for the 1990s. *Nature* 362.

Sircar, S., and U. Kansra. 1998. Choice of cooking oils—myths and realities. *Journal of the Indian Medical Association* 96(10).

Stanhope, J. M., Sampson V. M., Prior I. A. 1981. The Tokelau Island migrant study: Serum lipid concentrations in two environments. *Journal of Chronic Diseases* 34.

Thampan, P. K. 1994. *Facts and fallacies about coconut oil*. Jakarta: Asian and Pacific Coconut Community.

CHAPTER 4 • NATURE'S MARVELOUS GERM FIGHTER

Anonymous. 1987. Monolaurin. *AIDS Treatment News* 33.

Anonymous. 1998. Summertime blues: It's giardia season. *Journal of Environmental Health*, July/August 61.

Bergsson, G., Arnfinnsson S., Karlsson S. M., Steingrimsson O., Thormar H. 1998. In vitro inactivation of Chlamydia trachomatis by fatty acids and monoglycerides. *Antimicrobial Agents and Chemotherapy* 42.

Chowhan, G. S., Joshi K. R., Bhatnagar H. N., Khangarot D. 1985. Treatment of tapeworm infestation by coconut (*Concus nucifera*) preparations. *The Journal of the Association of Physicians of India* 33.

Crook, W. 1986. *The yeast connection*. New York: Vintage Books.

Crouch, A. A., Seow W. K., Whitman L. M., Thong Y. H. 1991. Effect of human milk and infant milk formulae on adherence of Giardia intestinalis. *Transactions of the Royal Society of Tropical Medicine and Hygiene* 85.

Enig, M. G. 1999. Coconut: In support of good health in the twenty-first century. Paper presented at the Thirty-sixth Annual Meeting of the APCC.

Food-borne illnesses a growing threat to public health. *American Medical News,* June 10, 1996.

Galland, L. 1999. Colonies within: Allergies from intestinal parasites. *Total Health* 21.

Galland, L., and M. Leem. 1990. *Giardia lamblia* infection as a cause of chronic fatigue. *Journal of Nutritional Medicine* 1.

Hernell, O., Ward H., Blackberg L., Pereira M. E. 1986. Killing of Giardia lamblia by human milk lipases: An effect mediated by lipolysis of milk lipids. *Journal of Infectious Diseases* 153.

Hierholzer, J. C., and J. J. Kabara. 1982. In vitro effects of monolaurin compounds on enveloped RNA and DNA viruses. *Journal of Food Safety* 4.

Holland, K. T., Taylor D., Farrell A. M. 1994. The effect of glycerol monolaurate on growth of, and production of toxic shock syndrome toxin-1 and lipase by, Staphylococcus aureus. *Journal of Antimicrobial Chemotherapy* 33.

Isaacs, C. E., and H. Thormar. 1991. The role of milk-derived antimicrobial lipids as antiviral and antibacterial agents. In *Immunology of milk and the neonate,* edited by J. Mestecky, Blair C., and Ogra P. L. New York: Plenum Press.

Isaacs, C. E., Litov R. E., Marie P., Thormar H. 1992. Addition of lipases to infant formulas produces antiviral and antibacterial activity. *Journal of Nutritional Biochemistry* 3.

Isaacs, C. E., Kim K. S., Thormar H. 1994. Inactivation of enveloped viruses in human bodily fluids by purified lipid. *Annals of the New York Academy of Sciences* 724.

Kabara, J. J. 1978. Fatty acids and derivatives as antimicrobial agents. In *The pharmacological effect of lipids,* edited by J. J. Kabara. Champaign, Ill.: American Oil Chemists' Society.

Kabara, J. J. 1984. Antimicrobial agents derived from fatty acids. *Journal of the American Oil Chemists Society* 61.

Merewood, A. 1994. Taming the yeast beast. *Women's Sports and Fitness* 16.

Novotny, T. E., Hopkins R. S., Shillam P., Janoff E. N. 1990. Prevalence of Giardia lamblia and risk factors for infection among children attending day-care. *Public Health Reports* 105.

Petschow, B. W., Batema R. P., Ford L. L. 1996. Susceptibility of Helicobacter pylori to bactericidal properties of medium-chain monoglycerides and free fatty acids. *Antimicrobial Agents and Chemotherapy* 145.

Reiner, D. S., Wang C. S., Gillin F. D. 1986. Human milk kills Giardia lamblia by generating toxic lipolytic products. *Journal of Infectious Diseases* 154.

Thormar, H., Isaacs C. E., Brown H. R., Barshatzky, M. R., Pessolano T. 1987. Inactivation enveloped viruses and killing of cells by fatty acids and monoglycerides. *Antimicrobial Agents and Chemotherapy* 31.

Wan, J. M., and R. F. Grimble. 1987. Effect of dietary linoleate content on the metabolic response of rats to *Escherichia coli* endotoxin. *Clinical Science* 72(3).

CHAPTER 5 • EAT FAT, LOSE WEIGHT

Baba, N. 1982. Enhanced thermogenesis and diminished deposition of fat in response to overfeeding with diet containing medium-chain triglyceride. *American Journal of Clinical Nutrition* 35.

Bray, G. A., Cee M., Bray T. L. 1980. Weight gain of rats fed medium-chain triglycerides is less than rats fed long-chain triglycerides. *International Journal of Obesity* 4.

Divi, R. L., Chang H. C., Doerge D. R. 1997. Anti-thyroid isoflavones from soybean: Isolation, characterization, and mechanisms of action. *Biochemical Pharmacology* 54(10).

Geliebter, A. 1980. Overfeeding with a diet containing medium chain triglyceride impedes accumulation of body fat. *Clinical Research* 28.

Geliebter, A., Torbay N., Bracco E. F., Hashim S. A., Van Itallie T. B. 1983. Overfeeding with medium-chain triglycerides diet results in diminished deposition of fat. *American Journal of Clinical Nutrition* 37.

Hasihim, S. A., and P. Tantibhedyangkul. 1987. Medium chain triglyceride in early life: Effects on growth of adipose tissue. *Lipids* 22.

Hill, J. O., Peters J. C., Yang D., Sharp T., Kaler M., Abumrad N. N., Greene H. L. 1989. Thermogenesis in humans during overfeeding with medium-chain triglycerides. *Metabolism* 38.

Ingle, D. L. 1999. Dietary energy value of medium-chain triglycerides. *Journal of Food Science* 64(6).

Murray, M. T. 1996. Herbal formulas containing natural sources of caffeine and ephedrine. *American Journal of Natural Medicine* 3(3).

Seaton, T. B., Welle S. L., Warenko M. K., Campbell R. G. 1986. Thermic effect of medium-chain and long-chain triglycerides in man. *American Journal of Clinical Nutrition* 44.

Shepard, T. H. 1960. Soybean goiter. *New England Journal of Medicine* 262.

Thampan, P. K. 1994. *Facts and fallacies about coconut oil.* Jakarta: Asian and Pacific Coconut Community.

Whitney, E. N., Cataldo C. B., Rolfes S. R. 1991. *Understanding normal and clinical nutrition.* 3rd ed. St. Paul, Minn.: West.

CHAPTER 6 • BEAUTIFUL SKIN AND HAIR

Anonymous. 1999. Shine to dye for. *Redbook,* February.

Cross, C. E., Halliwell B., Borish E. T., Pryor W. A., Ames B. N., Saul R. L., McCord J. M., Harman D. 1987. Oxygen radicals and human disease. *Annals of Internal Medicine* 107.

Harman, D. 1986. Free radical theory of aging: Role of free radicals in the origination and evolution of life, aging, and disease processes. In *Free radicals, aging and degenerative diseases,* edited by R. L. Walford, J. E. Johnson, D. Harman, and J. Miguel. New York: John Wiley & Sons.

Kabara, J. J. 1978. *The pharmacological effect of lipids.* Champaign, Ill.: The American Oil Chemists' Society.

Noonan, P. 1994. Porcupine antibiotics. *Omni* 16.

Sadeghi, S., Wallace F. A., Calder P .C. 1999. Dietary lipids modify the cytokine response to bacterial lipopolysaccharide in mice. *Immunology* 96(3).

CHAPTER 7 • COCONUT OIL AS FOOD AND AS MEDICINE

Anonymous. 1999. Low-fat diet alone reversed type 2 diabetes in mice. *Comprehensive Therapy* 25(1).

Campbell-Falck, D., Thomas T., Falck T. M., Tutuo N., Clem K. 2000. The intravenous of coconut water. *American Journal of Emergency Medicine* Jan: 18(1).

Applegate, L. 1996. Nutrition. *Runner's World* 31.

Azain, M. J. 1993. Effects of adding medium-chain triglycerides to sow diets during late gestation and early lactation on litter performance. *Journal of Animal Science* 71(11).

Balzola, F. A., Castellino F., Colombatto P., Manzini P., Astegiano M., Verme G., Brunetto M. R., Pera A., Bonino F. 1997. IgM antibody against measles virus in patients with inflammatory bowel disease: A marker of virus-related disease? *European Journal of Gastroenterology & Hepatology* 9(7).

Barnard, R. J., Massey M. R., Cherry S., O'Brien L. T., Pritikin, N. 1983. Long-term use of a high-complex-carbohydrate, high-fiber, low-fat diet and exercise in the treatment of NIDDM patients. *Diabetes Care* 6(3).

Berry, E. M. 1997. Dietary fatty acids in the management of diabetes mellitus. *American Journal of Clinical Nutrition* 66 (supp.).

Cha, Y. S., and D. S. Sachan. 1994. Opposite effects of dietary saturated and unsaturated fatty acids on ethanol-pharmacokinetics, triglycerides and carnitines. *Journal of the American College of Nutrition* 13(4).

Cohen, L. A. 1988. Medium chain triglycerides lack tumor-promoting effects in the n-methylnitrosourea-induced mammary tumor model. In *The pharmacological effects of lipids,* vol. 3, edited by J. J. Kabara. Champaign, Ill.: The American Oil Chemists' Society.

Cohen, L. A., and D. O. Thompson. 1987. The influence of dietary medium chain triglycerides on rat mammary tumor development. *Lipids* 22(6).

Daszak, P. 1997. Detection and comparative analysis of persistent measles virus infection in Crohn's disease by immunogold electron microscopy. *Journal of Clinical Pathology* 50(4).

Dayrit, C. S. 2000. Coconut oil in health and disease: Its and monolaurin's potential as cure for HIV/AIDS. Paper presented at the Thirty-seventh Annual Cocotech Meeting, Chennai, India, July 25.

Francois, C. A., Connor S. L., Wander R. L., Connor W .E. 1998. Acute effects of dietary fatty acids on the fatty acids of human milk. *American Journal of Clinical Nutrition* 67.

Fushiki, T., and K. Matsumoto. 1995. Swimming endurance capacity of mice is increased by chronic consumption of medium-chain triglycerides. *Journal of Nutrition* 125.

Garfinkel, M., Cee S., Opara E. C., Akwari O. E. 1992. Insulinotropic potency of lauric acid: A metabolic rationale for medium chain fatty acids (MCF) in TPN formulation. *Journal of Surgical Research* 52.

Ginsberg, B. H., Jabour J., Spector A. A. 1982. Effect of alterations in membrane lipid unsaturation on the properties of the insulin receptor of Ehrlich ascites cells. *Biochimica et biophysica acta* 690(2).

Goldberg, B., ed. 1994. *Alternative medicine.* Fife, Wash.: Future Medicine.

Hopkins, G. J., Kennedy T. G., Carroll K. K. 1981. Polyunsaturated fatty acids as promoters of mammary carcinogenesis induced in Sprague-Dawley rats by 7, 12-dimethylbenz[a]anthracene. *Journal of the National Cancer Institute* 66(3).

Jiang, Z. M., Zhang S. Y., Wang X. R. 1993. A comparison of medium-chain and long-chain triglycerides in surgical patients. *Annals of Surgery* 217(2).

Kiyasu, G. Y. 1952. The portal transport of absorbed fatty acids. *Journal of Biological Chemistry* 199.

Kono, H., Enomoto N., Connor H. D., Wheeler M. D., Bradford B. U., Rivera C. A., Kadiiska M. B., Mason R. P., Thurman R. G. 2000. Medium-chain triglycerides inhibit free radical formation and TNF-alpha production in rats given enteral ethanol. *American Journal of Physiology, Gastrointestinal and Liver Physiology* 278(3).

Lewin, J., Dhillon A. P., Sim R., Mazure G., Pounder R.E., Wakefield A. J. 1995. Persistent measles virus infection of the intestine: confirmation by immunogold electron microscopy. *Gut* 36(4).

Macalalag, E.V., Macalalag M. L., Macalalag A. L., Perez E. B., Cruz L. V., Valensuela L. S., Bustamante M. M., Macalalag M. E. 1997. Buko water of immature coconut is a universal urinary stone solvent. Paper presented at the Padivid Coconut Community Conference, Manila, August 14–18.

Monserrat, A. J., Romero M., Lago N., Aristi C. 1995. Protective effect of coconut oil on renal necrosis occurring in rats fed a methyl-deficient diet. *Renal Failure* 17(5).

Montgomery, S. M., Morris D. L., Pounder R. E., Wakefield A. J. 1999. Paramyxovirus infections in childhood and subsequent inflammatory bowel disease. *Gastroenterology* 116(4).

Murray, M. 1994. *Natural alternatives to over-the-counter and prescription drugs.* New York: Morrow.

Nanji, A. A., Sadrzadeh S. M., Yang E. K., Fogt F., Meydani M., Dannenberg A. J. 1995. Dietary saturated fatty acids: A novel treatment for alcoholic liver disease. *Gastroenterology* 109(2).

Oakes, N. D., Bell K. S., Furler S. M., Camilleri S., Saha A. K., Ruderman N. B., Chisholm D. S., Kraegen E. W. 1997. Diet-induced muscle insulin resistance in rats is ameliorated by acute dietary lipid withdrawal or a single bout of exercise: Parallel relationship between insulin stimulation of glucose uptake and suppression of long-chain fatty acyl-CoA. *Diabetes* 46(12).

Parekh, P. I., Petro A. E., Tiller J. M., Feinglos M. N., Surwit R. S. 1998. Reversal of diet-induced obesity and diabetes in C57BL/6J mice. *Metabolism* 47(9).

Reddy, B. S. 1992. Dietary fat and colon cancer: Animal model studies. *Lipids* 27(10).

Ross, D. L., Swaiman K. F., Torres F., Hansen J. 1985. Early biochemical and EEG correlates of the ketogenic diet in children with atypical absence epilepsy. *Pediatric Neurology* 1(2).

Shimada, H., Tyler V. E., McLaughlin J. L. 1997. Biologically active acylglycerides from the berries of saw-palmetto. *Journal of National Products* 60.

Sircar, S., and U. Kansra. 1998. Choice of cooking oils—myths and realities. *Journal of the Indian Medical Association* 96(10).

Tantibhedhyangkul, P., and S. A. Hashim. 1978. Medium-chain triglyceride feeding in premature infants: Effects on calcium and magnesium absorption. *Pediatrics* 61(4).

Thampan, P. K. 1994. *Facts and fallacies about coconut oil.* Jakarta: Asian and Pacific Coconut Community.

Vaidya, U. V., Hegde V. M., Bhave S. A., Pandit A. N. 1992 Vegetable oil fortified feeds in the nutrition of very low birthweight babies. *Indian Pediatrics* 29(12).

Wakefield, A. J., Montgomery S. M., Pounder R. E. 1999. Crohn's disease: The case for measles virus. *Italian Journal of Gastroenterology and Hepatology* 31(3).

Watkins, B. A. 2000. Importance of vitamin E in bone formation and in chondroncyte function, Purdue University. Cited in S. Fallon and M. G.

Enig, Dem bones—do high protein diets cause osteoporosis? *Wise Traditions* 1(4).

Yost, T. J., and R. H. Eckel. 1989. Hypocaloric feeding in obese women: Metabolic effects of medium-chain triglyceride substitution. *American Journal of Clinical Nutrition* 49(2).

CHAPTER 8 • EAT YOUR WAY TO BETTER HEALTH

Gerster, H. 1998. Can adults adequately convert alpha-linolenic acid (18:3n-3) to eicosapentaenoic acid (20:5n-3) and docosahexaenoic acid (22:6n-3)? *International Journal for Vitamin and Nutrition Research* 68(3).

Isaacs, C. E., and H. Thormar. 1990. Human milk lipids inactivated enveloped viruses. In *Breastfeeding, nutrition, infection and infant growth in developed and emerging countries,* edited by S. A. Atkinson, L. A. Hanson, and R. K. Chandra. St. John's, Newfoundland: Arts Biomedical.

Kabara, J. J. 1984. Laurcidin: The nonionic emulsifier with antimicrobial properties. In *Cosmetic and drug perservation, principles and practice,* edited by Jon J. Kabara. New York: Marcel Dekker.

Traul, K. A., Driedger A., Ingle D. L., Nakhasi D. 2000. Review of the toxicologic properties of medium-chain triglycerides. *Food and Chemical Toxicology* 38(1).

World Health Organization/Food and Agriculture Organization. 1977. *Dietary fats and oils in human nutrition.* Report of an expert consultation. Rome: U.N. Food and Agriculture Organization.

INDEX

ABOUT THE AUTHOR

Dr. Bruce Fife, C.N., N.D., is an author, speaker, certified nutritionist, and naturopath. He has written 18 books, including *Eat Fat, Look Thin,* and *Coconut Lover's Cookbook*. He is the director of the southern Colorado chapter of the Weston A. Price Foundation, a nonprofit organization dedicated to nutritional education. He is the publisher and editor of the *Healthy Ways Newsletter*. He serves as the president of the Coconut Research Center, an organization whose purpose is to educate the public about the health and nutritional aspects of coconut.

He was the first to gather together the medical research on the health benefits of coconut oil and present it in an understandable and readable format for the general public. Because of this, he is recognized as one of the leading authorities on the health benefits of coconut oil. For this reason he is often referred to as the "Coconut Guru," and many respectfully call him "Dr. Coconut."